NEURO-SEMANTICS

The Book

Actualizing

Your Highest Meanings

and Best Performances

L. Michael Hall, Ph.D.

© **2011** **Neuro-Semantics:**
Actualizing Meaning and Performance
L. Michael Hall, Ph.D.
Library of Congress, Washington, D.C., Copyright Pending

ISBN

ISBN 978-189000140-7

9 781890 001407

90000

Published by: **NSP** —*Neuro-Semantics Publications*
P.O. Box 8
Clifton, CO. 81520-0008 USA
(970) 523-7877

Neuro-Semantics® is the trademark name for the model, patterns, and
society of Neuro-Semantics. ISNS stands for the International Society of
Neuro-Semantics. For more than 5000 pages of free information, see the
web sites:

www.neurosemantics.com
www.meta-coaching.org
www.self-actualizing.org
www.nlp-video.com — **www.ns-video.com**

Neuro-Semantics

1: What is Neuro-Semantics?   1

A description of what Neuro-Semantics means, list of elements in the model, and a description of the Neuro-Semantic model in terms of its key premises.

Part I: The Dimension of Meaning

2: Meaning-Making — The Human Adventure   22

A description of how meaning-making works from the unspeakable level to the level of association as you become conscious of our world and the things you are referring to. As you use experiences and events as references for how you think about it, you then bring that world inside to create representational meaning. You make meaning by creating frames—your internal contexts for understanding.

3: The Kinds of Meaning   42

The different kinds of meaning as well as the different levels of meaning, explains how you create your Matrix of Meaning Frames and the psycho-logical structures that emerge. Your meaning-making occurs in all of these different ways and yet these are just different descriptions, different maps about these things. Knowing all of this, you can now begin to simplify the complexity of your meaning system. All of this generates your unique Neuro-Semantic landscape.

4: The Levels of Meaning   61

There are levels of meaning—meaning-making moves from the primary level to the layering of meanings upon meanings. Using your self-reflexive consciousness, you create logical levels which are actually not so logical, but psycho-logical. You can discover these levels via the meta-questions.

Part II: The Performance of Meaning   151

you set frames and reframe. Framing lies at the core of all creativity. The semantic skills of inventing and re-constructing meaning describes what it means to be human.

Meaning often hides in stories— the stories that have been told you about you, your family, your background. And as a form of meaning— some stories are toxically limiting. So enacting meaning often takes the form of narrating a new story that you then tell yourself and others which you can then embody as a new way of being in the world.

Since we negotiate meaning and do so via communicating with ourselves and others, as you learn how to actualize your own communication excellence, you access and use the highest of your meaning-making skills. There *communion* occurs. Then you connect and raise the quality of the relationship.

The ultimate in meaning-making is to identify and create meanings that enable you and others to perform *excellence*. Where there are best practices or human experiences of excellence, there is a structure. And where there is a dynamic structure of meaning and frames— we can identify them and replicate them to pass on the excellence.

If you want to grow up to become a competent Neuro-Semanticist, here are some of the required insights and skills you'll need.

INTRODUCTION

"Only to the extent to which man fulfills a meaning
out there in the world, does he fulfill himself."
Viktor Frankl (1969)

This is a book about Neuro-Semantics. I first began thinking about writing this in 1994 when I discovered and formulated the Meta-States Model. But I wasn't ready then; the model wasn't ready at that time. In 1994 I could *not* have written it. And so I did not! The model has taken nearly two decades to develop and evolve to become what it is today. It has taken that amount of time for application of the model, testing where it works and where it does not, and continuing research for further development. Now, nearly two decades later, I am beginning to be able to describe what Neuro-Semantics is.

Yet in saying that statement, I know that Neuro-Semantics is not finished. There is so much more to be developed in Neuro-Semantics in the coming decades in terms of patterns and applications. The discovery of meaning-making to actualize our highest and best has just begun. We have just touched the hem of the garment.

Actually, the models-yet-to-be-developed could very well make redundant many of the patterns or even the models in this book. And that's okay. That has happened in many other fields. It happened in NLP. And if Neuro-Semantics continues to be a dynamic and ever-evolving field, then that will be a sign of growth as fresh new models and patterns are created and innovated.

I have divided this book into two parts. First, *the dimension of meaning* and then second, *the performance of meaning.* That's because as of this date (2011), one of the most basic Neuro-Semantic models is the Meaning— Performance Axes. The first part is mostly theoretical; it provides the premises and understandings for the Neuro-Semantic Models. The second part is mostly practical; it provides specific things you can do to enrich the quality of your meanings. There you'll find two dozen patterns for your neuro-semantic development.

What ties meaning and performance together? *Self-Actualization.* That's why self-actualization is a function of your highest meanings and your best performances. This solves the mind-body dichotomy. Now you can see that these are two functions of the same thing. Your neurology, out of which you perform, and your semantics from which you meanings and meaning-making define your actions, when these two functions come together they generate your neuro-semantic states and reality. Doing this simultaneously closes your knowing–doing.

Neuro-Semantics is a very dynamic model precisely because it is systemic. As a systemic model it embraces both sides of the old dichotomy and holds them together. Your semantics are *not* distinct from or separate from your neurology, physiology, or physical states. Your semantics are intimately embodied in your moment-to-moment states. Your semantics are expressed at any given moment in your emotions, your moods, your attitudes, your expressions verbally and behaviorally. Your semantics also originate and are created within the context of your functioning nervous systems (your neurology). It is all inter-related.

Is this a difficult book? Is it a highly academic work? The short answer is *No.* The longer answer is that it is also not a shallow, quick-to-read book. I have sought to make it as simple as I can without over-simplifying it.

Did I create this book by cutting-and-pasting materials from previously written books? No. At least 95 per cent of the book is freshly written and *not* merely copied. I was particularly conscious of this when I started. So rather than make it a collection of previously published materials, I sat down and wrote the first draft completely afresh. Only later did I compare what

I wrote here with other writings, and on occasion I did fill in details from things that I had previously written. Yet as you read, you will see diagrams that have been used before and some stories previously told. The design throughout has been to write in a way that meets two criteria—to be complete and thorough— to be fresh and easy to read.

My design in this book is also to pull together the central essence of Neuro-Semantics and to identify all of the models within this field at this date. Doing this will provide a map of the landscape of Neuro-Semantics and enable you as a reader to identify the areas of particular interest to you.

Is Neuro-Semantics a new psychology? No. It is however a new synthesis of several psychologies and several philosophies which makes it truly an inter-disciplinary model. The psychologies it embraces are: Cognitive, Behavioral, Existential, Developmental, Humanistic or Self-Actualization Psychology. The philosophies it operates from include: Phenomenology General Semantics, Cognitive Linguistics, etc.

Welcome to the Neuro-Semantic adventure!

Chapter 1

WHAT IS

NEURO-SEMANTICS?

"Neuro-Semantics: Taking NLP to a higher level
professionally and ethically."
L. Michael Hall, 1996 Original Vision Statement

Everyday someone asks me, *"What is Neuro-Semantics?"* And every time I'm asked, I am tempted to look at my watch to see how much time I have to answer that question. I could easily and quickly say, "It's your neurology and your meanings; it's your embodied meanings that comprise your life and that create what for you makes sense in life." And while that is true, it is also superficial. Neuro-Semantics is so much more.

Neuro-Semantics is the exploration of meaning (semantics) and how we humans, as meaning-makers, make meaning. Exploring the structure of meaning and how we construct, construe, and interpret the events of life endowing them with meaning, Neuro-Semantics focuses on expanding the ability to detect meaning frames, the processes of meaning-making, quality controlling meanings, enriching limiting meaning, suspending dis-empowering meanings, and taking charge of one's meaning-making instinct. So *Neuro-Semantics,* as a mind-body-emotion discipline, refers to how we human beings create, experience, and transform *meaning* within their bodies as performances (actions, skills, gestures, etc.).

Neuro-Semantics goes beyond merely exploring meaning, it enables the skills of meaning-making. It especially enables the processes of identifying meaningful possibilities that represent your highest visions and values in life and actualizing those potentials in your best performance in everyday life to achieve your highest goals and dreams.

Neuro-Semantics is a practical set of processes for unleashing your highest and best and actualizing them so that your life is richly meaningful and significant. In this unleashing, there is an unleashing *from* the things that limit, interfere, and sabotage your best and an unleashing *to* your dreams of a highly productive and meaningful life. We call this unleashing process—self-actualization.

Neuro-Semantics is *a communication model* for exploring how the *body* (neuro-, the nervous system, physiology, neurology) gets *programmed* by the use of *language* (linguistics, symbols), and *meaning* (semantics). NLP focuses on the linear and horizontal tracking of the processes of the mind. NLP focuses on the **how** of human behavior. Its central question is, "How do you do that behavior?" Neuro-Semantics adds another distinction—the **why** of behavior (its meaning). From a higher level of mind, *meaning* drives behavior. There are many hidden *meta* (Greek for "above and about") levels of thought and meaning within the structure of subjective experience.

Neuro-Semantics is a positive, strength-based psychology designed to model the highest and best in human nature so we can transfer it to our everyday lives. The tag-line of Neuro-Semantics, *Actualizing Excellence,* identifies that we primarily model expertise and best practices. We are able to do this because every experience has a structure. Sometimes we also model dysfunctional experiences to understand how diminishing experiences work. Knowing how an experience works enables us to be able to transform it for higher purposes.

Neuro-Semantics is an expression of the positive psychology that Maslow and Rogers pioneered (Humanistic, Self-Actualization Psychology) that gave birth to NLP and dozens of other strength-based psychologies. In recovering its original NLP history, Neuro-Semantics is rediscovering the health-based philosophy that focuses on the further reaches of human nature.

There you have it! Six paragraphs that define and map out Neuro-Semantics. And I'm sure that with these descriptions, you now have many more questions about Neuro-Semantics. To answer those questions, I will identify the essential variables within Neuro-Semantics and then I'll set out a list of the fundamental premises that govern our activity as Neuro-Semanticists.

Chief Variables of the Neuro-Semantic Model
The definitions you just read identify several variables, elements, or components that stand out as central to the Neuro-Semantic model. When you know these seven key variables, you will have an even fuller description and understanding. So here goes:
- *1) Meaning*: Neuro-Semantics is all about meaning—what it is, how we call it into existence, how we create it, how we keep it within us, live it, embody it, how we can change it, suspend it, and even release it. When Korzybski said that we humans are a semantic-class of life he identified *meaning* as the key variable within our mind-body-emotion system that determines the conditions and quality of our life. This makes meaning absolutely crucial to how you experience life, your actions, relationships, and the significance of your life.

  Meaning is not a singular thing, nor is it a linear thing. In fact, it is not a *thing* at all. To speak of meaning as a noun (a nominalization) falsely betrays its true nature. *Meaning is a process*—it is something you and I *do*. We *make meaning*. And we do so in numerous ways. As you will learn, we make meaning via associating one thing with another so that they become linked and connected. The things don't have to be logically linked or connected. But link them, and you make that as your "meaning." This starts the journey into the fuzzy world where you can create all kinds of "logics" (reasonings).

- *2) Neurology*: It is by, and within, your nervous systems that you create meaning. Your neurology entails all of your nervous systems (central nervous system, autonomic, immune, sympathetic, parasympathetic, etc.). It also is part and parcel of your spinal chord and brain including all of the levels of your brain. Korzybski mapped the major components of the brain and identified the sequence of their functioning, how lower level impulses that enter into the brain at the thalamus and are processed by being sent to the higher levels. It is within the neurology of your body, physiology, neuro-chemistry, neuro-pathways, etc. that you construct and hold meaning. Mind-and-body together, as an integrated system, creates your neuro-semantic existence.

- *3) Performance*: From the interactions of your neuro-semantic mind-body-emotion system arise your internal behaviors as you *somatize your meanings* into your emotions, and then react, gesture, speak, and act. All of these behaviors, micro- and macro-, comprise the feed-forward loop of communication as you turn "information" or "data' about the world and yourself into actions. As a mind-body-emotion system, your life is a matter of *information into the system and energy out*. The energy out shows up as performance —this includes both actions that are healthy and effective and those that are neurotic and dysfunctional.

- *4) Development*: As a neuro-semantic class of life, at birth you are born only partially developed. Your brain does not fully develop until puberty when certain hormones facilitates the maturing of your physical brain. And from infancy to young adulthood, many of your semantic dimensions develop through stages that have been well-mapped out by Developmental Psychologists. During that period, you develop cognitively, socially, sexually, and ethically. As you develop through definite cognitive-emotional stages, if you evolve in a healthy way, you move beyond the cognitive distortions of childhood and discover how to effectively cope with your basic or lower needs. Abraham Maslow identified the mechanism of deficiency as the nature of these lower needs, and if you successfully evolve beyond the lower animal needs, you move to the truly human needs—the "self-actualization" needs that operate by the mechanism of abundance, *being-ness,* and meaningfulness.

• *5) Self-Actualization*: You are an evolutionary developmental class of life who develops by the effectiveness of your semantic mapping. First you have to create a mental model of what your needs are and how to fulfill them (chapter 9). Then you have to generate a mental model that allows you to learn, practice, and integrate accurate and effective ways to cope with those needs. Semantically coding your needs accurately brings true gratification so that you keep evolving to the next level of needs [survival, safety, social (love and affection), self, self-actualization]. That's when you semantically code the higher needs in a way that brings out your highest visions and values in life and transfer them to your best performances.

• *6) Inner and Outer Game*: A user-friendly way to talk about Neuro-Semantics is to speak the *inner game* of constructing your frames of meaning so that you have useful, actionable, and relevant mental models for how to cope with the demands of everyday life. This is what "learning" is all about—learning what things are, how they work, what they lead to, how they operate in social contexts, and how to cope with life's challenges. The inner game comes first because if your understandings, beliefs, decisions, identities, intentions, etc. are wrongly formatted, then your actions will fail you as you seek to navigate the territory to which they refer. Conversely, *the outer game* of effective actions that produce results in all of the dimensions of life indicate that you know, understand, and have an effective strategy for that domain.
Psycho-logics is the term that describes the unique meaning of your inner games. This term was created by Korzybski by hyphenating

the terms psychology and psychological. When you make meaning using your neuro-linguistic mind-body-emotion states, you create a world of meaning for yourself that is "psycho-logical." This means that from within the frames and references that you create about your world, *it all makes perfect sense.* It may not make useful, productive, or enhancing sense, but it makes "psycho-logical" sense as you have created a world of meaning by the way you reasoned.

As you *make meaning,* you do not do so only by associations and the wild forms of psycho-logics that emerge, but you do so mostly by how you *mentally frame* things. This refers to the higher forms of your meaning-making. You first link things, then you take that linkage inside yourself by *representing* it as a map of the external world. This representation operates as the way you "think"about something. Then some higher level "magic" occurs. You do not just represent things, you alter and play and manipulate and change the things you represent. You also then step back to think about those things again and again, layer upon layer. This creates higher level abstractions. And this process of reflexive thinking reflecting back onto your previous thoughts never ends. You can always think-feel about whatever you think.

As a symbolic class of life you use symbols to "stand for" things out there. Then you create symbols to stand for those symbols. This complicates things as you create internal contexts which you then use to understand and interpret things. As you create these layers of mental contexts (frames) you generate more complex conceptual understandings as your schemes and paradigms.

- *7) Modeling*: Given your neuro-semantic nature, the central key to successful navigating of the territory is finding, creating, designing, and installing an effective mental model. The process of doing that is called *modeling.* So Neuro-Semantics is a model of *how to model* experiences. Neuro-Semantics, following the pioneering modeling work of Maslow (Self-Actualization Psychology) and of Bandler and Grinder (Neuro-Linguistic Programming) is centrally about the modeling process (chapter 17). Primarily we model human excellence and expertise. We also can, and do, model dysfunctional experiences in order to understand the frames of meaning (beliefs, decisions, intentions, understandings, etc.) that make the dysfunctional experience work as it does. This informs us what to do to create generative change.

Neuro-Semantics provides flexible tools for tracking the vertical or higher dimensions of mental processing. It even provides models for tracking the systemic nature of mind as it moves round and round the circuits of ideas, memories, concepts, imaginations, etc. As a tool for more fully identifying the higher and ever-changing levels of human consciousness and meaning that drive behavior, Neuro-Semantics enables us to track, model, and replicate human excellence.

The Neuro-Semantic Model
With this list of variables that make up Neuro-Semantics, I am now able to describe the model itself. I will do so in a progressive way beginning with the elements of the model that are most obvious, overt, and explicit and move on to those that are more hidden, implicit, and unconscious.

Premise 1: Neuro-Semantics begins with neuro-semantic states. Almost any and every consideration about yourself or another person, or even a group as an organization of people, begins with state. You begin by considering a person's behaviors, linguistics, or emotions because these are expressions of state. They are the outward and external expressions of a person (or group of persons). And they come from a state— a mind-body-emotional state.

State, a key word in Neuro-Semantics and NLP, because it is *the grounding experience.* Whatever is going on in the mind, if it is real, if it is substantial, then it shows up in the person's mind-body-emotion state. This neuro-semantic and neuro-linguistic state is a systemic process of all of the person's thinking, framing, remembering, imaging, anticipating, hoping, fearing, believing, and so on. And while we can linguistically sort out some things as "mental" and some as "emotional," this artificial separating is only linguistic. In reality, mind-body, mental-emotional go together as a system.

State is a holistic or systemic term that captures the fullness of the experience more accurately.

Now regarding *state,* you and I and everybody and every group are always in a state. The question is not whether we are in a state, but *what state* are you in, how intense is the state, how pure, how mixed, how useful or unuseful, how resourceful or unresourceful, how much are you in control of the state or how much does the state have you?

In fact, exploring state with such questions explores the very territory that is covered by the Emotional Intelligence model (EQ). The EQ model uses a more dichotomous term ("emotion") and seeks to enable people to develop emotional awareness, monitoring, management, and use in relating. We do this in Neuro-Semantics explicitly by exploring what state, how intense, what triggers it, what intensifies or reduces it, how to anchor it, qualify it, and then use it for navigating the world.

Using the foundations of NLP, in Neuro-Semantics we recognize that you can access a state through memory ("Imagine a time when..."), imagination ("What would it be like if..."), or modeling ("Do you know anyone who experiences this..."). This gives us two royal roads into state— thinking and acting. By recalling and imagining you can get yourself into a state. You can also adopt the physiology characteristic of a state and in that way act your way into state. Both provide "emotional management" tools so that you can have the state rather than the state having you.

Anchoring a state, another NLP contribution, adapts Pavlov's discoveries that are used in Behaviorism, as a user-friendly way to work methodically with a state. By linking sensory-based trigger to a state, you can link that trigger (a sight, sound, smell, word, gesture, movement, etc.) to the state and thereby be able to elicit, increase, decrease, or alter the state so that it can work more effectively to enable a person to be more resourceful in responding to life's challenges.[1]

Premise 2: Neuro-Semantics ground neuro-semantic states. In working with human experiences, you not only have to identify the state that it comes from and the expressions that comes out of that state, you need to ground that state so that you can explore its depths and transform it. *Grounding a state* is critical because states, as processes, are forever moving, changing, and altering. You can and do shift states quickly and rapidly and unless you *ground* it, the very experience that you want to enrich, alter, transform, or use can disappear.

A state, as a process, *is a process of thinking, framing, believing, emoting, speaking, acting, moving, etc.* It is not a thing. It is not static. And as a system, anyone who enters that system *by the very act of making contact with it changes it.* There is no naive observer position. Every act of observation, noticing, witnessing, speaking, communicating, inter-acting, etc. *influences and affects* the mind-body-emotion system of the state. Hence the reason to ground the state.

Now grounding a state is an anchoring process. And with primary states, a sensory-based anchor is generally sufficient to ground it. Not so, however, with higher or meta-states. For those, the grounding process involves more.

Primary states refers to states that are thinking-framing-emoting responses to something or some person in the world. You are making a thinking-and-feeling response to something "out there." The referent is real, actual, and physical. *A higher or meta-state* refers to a state in which you are offering a thinking-framing-emoting response to a previous state. Now you are thinking-and-emoting *about* a thought, a feeling, a response. You are self-reflexively in response to yourself. It is your second thought-feeling to a first thought-feeling.

In a primary state you might think-and-feel *fear* about a barking dog, closed space, high cliff, snake, etc. In a meta-state, you are thinking-and-feeling *shame* about your *fear,* or *fear of your fear,* or *anger at your fear,* or *curiosity about your fear,* or even *pride of your fear.* In the higher state about a state, your focus is not on a thing, person, or event "out there." You are now focused on what's occurring "within" yourself. And this self-reflexive process is an infinite process so that you will also respond to your meta-response: *depressed* about your *fear* of your *fear.* And, in fact, with each response, you can respond yet again and do so without end. You can always step back to respond with another state to the previous state or states.[2]

To *ground* a meta-state, you have to repeat back and get a confirmation from the person about his or her thinking-feeling states. And doing that feeding-back and confirming begins to *hold* the meta-state in place in the person's mind so that you can then work with the meta-stating structure. Knowing that none of this is a "thing," that none of this is externally real, and that you as a visitor are influencing and inviting change by your very presence heightens your understanding of the importance of the grounding process.

Premise 3: Neuro-Semantics invites a mindfulness by accessing of your self-reflexive consciousness. The reason for the grounding is so that you can hold the experience stable as you explore it. Without the grounding, the experience itself easily morphs into other experiences and the person can start a negative downward spiraling that will make things worse. I'm speaking here of working with another person because it is far easier at first to work with another person, or have someone else work with you, than to do this with yourself.

There's a reason: Your self-reflexive consciousness. If your *neuro-semantic states* were only composed of one layer and you could just think of one thing at a time, it would be pretty easy to stay focused, not get side-tracked, and not get into spin. But minds are not so simple. You do not just think or just feel. You think-feel about your thinking-and-feeling and do so in a nano-second, layer upon layer. You do not just process information and make an internal movie with your thoughts of what you see, hear, sense, smell, taste, and say. You reflect upon whatever you experience and do so repeatedly.

It is your self-reflexive consciousness that is your greatest glory and deepest agony. With it you can ascend to the highest visions and values and dreams possible and feel an ecstasy and delight in just thinking-emoting about something. And with it also you can create internal nightmares that distance you from reality, distort the messages you send to your body, and that drive you insane so that you become a danger to yourself and others.

The Meta-States Model in Neuro-Semantics is the model that enables you to appreciate, understand, and work with your *reflexivity.* This dynamic, systemic process distinguishes you from all of the animals and makes our kind of consciousness so special, so incredibly powerful, so sacred, and so dangerous. Without the ability to recognize and manage the reflexivity, you can get yourself into a spin that can diminish you as a human being and even make you a candidate for suicide. The way you respond to your responses can become so toxic, so perditious, and so morbid that you become your own worst enemy as you just sit and "think."[3]

Yet your reflexivity is precisely the mechanism that also enables you to transcend and include your previous states. *Within the reflexivity process is your power of transcendence*—you can transcend any current reality. You can transcend and escape, you can transcend and build masterful resources into yourself and your states, you can transcend what *is* and begin to create what *can be,* you can transcend difficulties and problems and invent incredible solutions that only are available to those who can access the unimaginable potentials of human beings.

It is your self-reflexive consciousness that lies at the heart of all "spiritual" states and that expands consciousness so that you are not limited merely to the past, to what has been, but you can imagine new possibilities and then reverse engineer unimaginable solutions. It is this reflexivity that lies at the heart of science, human improvement, the dreams and visions and values that make all of us "religious" at heart. No wonder it is imperative that we take charge of this reflexivity and learn to manage it effectively!

Premise 4: Neuro-Semantics invites and provides direction for how to explore higher neuro-semantics states. So how do you get there? How do you rise above your first-level primary states and enter into the human experience of these layers upon layers of meta-states? How do you go about exploring the meta-levels of the mind so that you can now enter into a person's inner world more deeply?

Begin with rapport skills of NLP. Listen for the specific words and expressions that a person offers. Watch for and detect her specific ways of gesturing and using her body and then feed that information back, become a living, breathing bio-feedback mirror to the person. Do this in an attitude of respect, care, and sensitivity, and you create the experience of "rapport" or trust with that person. Doing that typically creates the sense of safety with you so that you earn the right to enter into that person's inner world of meanings.

The structure and strategy of rapport as discovered in NLP involves matching and mirroring the outputs of a person— the energy that they express in their speech and behavior. You receive it at the primary level and mirror it back. As you then enter in further and further, you continue to repeat this same process. As you hear meta-level expressions— value words, idiosyncratic expressions, beliefs, etc., you simply mirror it back as expressions of those higher states, invite the person to confirm or disconfirm, and hold it for them.

In this way, the receiving the person's feedback and mirroring back (giving it back) makes you a living, breathing bio-feedback mirror which enables the person to *hold* and *ground* the experience. Typically, doing this rather than problem-solving, giving advice, lecturing, teaching, correcting, etc., is so new and strange that it is a incredible and marvelous experience that for the first time enables the person is really able to see, hold, and embrace oneself. And with that, both you and them can then move up to the next level. Now the exploration has truly begun.[4]

This is why the first step in any communication with another human being has to be listening, questioning, exploring, checking out, reflecting back, and suspending judgment to enter into that person's world. If you don't do that, you can't even begin to "understand" the meanings that drive and govern that person's experiences. This "pacing" involves using all of your *output systems* (not only your words, but our postures, movements, tones, etc.) to match or fit in with the person you're communicating with.

To *pace* in that way is the basis for mutual understanding. It enables you to enter into the other person's *structured* reality. It gives you a way to try on another reality structure. When you do that from a stance of respect for the person, a desire to truly understand and to help, the person feels understood, confirmed, and validated. You don't have to agree with the other person in order to create such strong and powerful subjective experiences, you only have to *match the other's experience of the world.* Doing so gives you entrance.

Then, from there you earn the right to *lead* them somewhere else. You can influence them in ways that will enrich and enhance their experience. This holds true whether you are a formal change agent like therapist, hypnotist, teacher, marketer, manager, sales person, or less direct influencers— a lover, parent, friend, etc.[5]

By receiving whatever the person says and respecting it as that person's mental model of the world, and by not judging or evaluating it, but just hearing it, that *enables them to also hear it.* And whatever they offer you, whatever they say is just words, just gestures, just emotions. And it is real to them. It may not be real to you. It may not make sense to you. That's besides the point. The exploration is not about you! You don't have to agree in order to understand. You only have to hold this space and let them go into the next higher level of their mind.

The next higher level is a layer of thought-and-feeling which operates as a frame. Its position, as a context for thinking and interpreting, makes it a frame of meaning or a frame of mind. And as such, it makes up the Matrix of frames that the person lives inside of. And from inside it is *psychological*. Whenever or however the person drew the conclusions and made the interpretations that created that layer of thoughts-and-feelings, it made sense to them at that time. Of course, it could have been created by a 15-year old brain or a 5 year old brain or even a 9-month old brain and so may be childish, ridiculous, wrong, even stupid. Yet when created, it made sense and continues to make sense until seen, examined, and then changed.

Frames of reference which you and I experience as our frames of mind or frames of meaning are like that. Regardless of your age or mental capacity or life circumstances, when you take a referent event that happens to you and *represent* it within your mind (re-present it to yourself as your thought) you thereby *hold* it in mind. That is what the term "meaning" means— "to hold in mind." So whatever you hold in mind is what something means to you.

This explains how you can get some really stupid, toxic, childish, and accidental meanings lodged in your mind as your frames of reference. Some event happens and it catches your attention, it triggers a strong emotional state, and so you *bring it in by representing it in the theater of your mind.* Then you don't let it go. Instead you reflect upon it. And yes, you may reflect on it with a 3-year old mind! You draw conclusions, you make interpretations, decisions, beliefs, understandings, identities, etc. You layer thought-and-feeling layer upon layer building up a whole matrix of frames about that event. And given the primitive cognitive style of thinking during infancy and childhood, it's no wonder that you create all sorts of limiting, stupid, and even toxic ideas about things, about the world, about yourself, about others.

Now unless there are been plenty of corrective experiences or unless you have engaged in a self-awareness program to chase out the limiting beliefs, like most people you probably have lots of limiting frames at the top of your Matrix of frames. And most of them are outside-of-conscious awareness. These are your unquestioned assumptions that organize your perceptions and responses and that make up your inner reality. If you were conscious of them, your very consciousness of them would cause many of them to just vanish away. But you are not conscious of them. They make up your blind-spots. So they operate as your unconscious, assumptive presuppositions about life. And that's what makes them powerful and dangerous.

This highlights a central Neuro-Semantic distinction: *Higher levels govern the lower levels of thought and meaning.* And that leads to a key principle: Personal effectiveness is about utilizing and using these higher meta-levels of mind. The best and most pervasive personal change is made at these higher levels of mind. And here lies the difference that makes a difference.

Neuro-Semantics enables you to look at the frames of reference you use to make sense of things. Frames grow from how you take a reference event "out there," bring it into your mind, represent it, use it as a map, and then transform it into a frame of reference, frame of

> *Higher levels govern the lower levels of thought and meaning.*

mind, and the frameworks of your conceptual understandings.   "Mind" grows in this way. It evolves and transforms and emerges from within your neuro-linguistic system. And just when you have it mapped, it changes.

To tolerate the journey around the loops of reflexivity and up and down the embedded frames within frames, you have to have a good stomach for putting up with ambiguity, paradox, uncertainty, transitions, and transcendence.

Premise 5: Neuro-Semantics de-mystifies many of the old myths of psychology and philosophy. Recognizing this structure of mental-emotional frames demystifies a lot in human psychology. First and foremost it clarifies that there's nothing wrong with you. If you have a problem—the problem lies in your frames, not in you. This specifies another one of our key premises in Neuro-Semantics (#1): *The person is never the problem; the frame is the problem.*

Another demystification is this (#2): *There is nothing inside you but frames and frames are made out of images, sounds, sensations, and words.* There's nothing alien within you which needs to be cast out. The worst experiences of a human being— the personality dis-orderings are just that, *the dis-ordering* of a person's thinking-and-feeling. The person is not flawed or broken or sick, the person is suffering from flawed and sick frames. That's why exorcism isn't called for, education is. What is needed is a renewal of the mind and the transformation of the governing frames.[6]

Anther de-mystification (#3): *There is a structure that makes psycho-logical sense of every experience.* It all makes sense! Well, it makes sense *from the inside.* It makes sense given the frames that any person is living within. If I had those frames, I'd be thinking and feeling and believing and acting as the person who has these frames. And because it makes sense, because there is a structure that we can identify and make explicit— transformation involves changing the frames. It is as simple as that; it is as profound as that.

De-mystification #4: *Human nature can be changed and that change can be without pain.* Two of the old ideas are first, "You can't

> *The person is never the problem; the frame is the problem.*

change human nature," and second, "Change is hard and painful and takes a long time." These statements were indeed true given the tools that mankind has had for most of its history. They were even true through the early years of psychotherapy. Yet with the tools that are now available in Neuro-Semantics, we have made these old belief statements redundant. After all, if the problem is the frame, not the person, we do not have to fight or wrestle or trick the person. Instead we can align with the person and facilitate the person changing his or her own frames. That's because we can change no one, but we can facilitate any person to choose to make changes which he or she wants to make.

Premise 6: Neuro-Semantics searches for the structure of experiences.
Neuro-Semantics arose from the revolutionary work of Alfred Korzybski in the field of General Semantics via his book *Science and Sanity.* That work initiated the search for structure. That's because Korzybski said that *the only content of knowledge is structure.* If our maps are not *the same* as the territory, but are symbols, maps, representations, facsimiles of the territory, then *structure*, and structure only, can give clue as to what we're dealing with and how to cope effectively as we move through the territory.

From this concept Korzybski provides NLP its foundation. The developers of NLP founded their approach upon the core principle of General Semantics: *"The map is not the territory."* That lead them to searching for the *structure* of the interventions and communications that seemed so magical which that they found in the therapeutic geniuses—Fritz Perls, Virginia Satir, and Milton Erickson. And with the development of NLP, of "the study of the structure of subjectivity," came a whole field dedicated to modeling the structure of experience.[7]

In the meantime, other disciplines developed a very similar vision and direction. From the Cognitive Sciences, the neuro-sciences, meta-cognition, cognitive linguistics, artificial intelligence, etc., the search for structure continued.

Neuro-Semantics, growing out of NLP and other disciplines, continues this adventure of studying the structure of intentionality and meaning. Doing this takes NLP to a new level. Using *the Meta-States Model,* we explore *the levels of mind* to model the systemic structure we find in actual awareness. This means modeling the structure of reflexivity, recursiveness, thinking in circles, thinking in loops, going round and round, etc. It's all very messy. It lacks the nice linear black-and-white structure of Behaviorism's old Stimulus—Response model.

Premise 7: Neuro-Semantics facilitates the change process in multiple ways. I have already mentioned three change factors: create a high quality relationship of rapport for the safety and trust that allows a person to experience a mirroring of his or her own reality. The older psychologists (Freud, Adler, Jung, etc.) often said, "Awareness *per se* is curative." And sometimes it is. Sometimes when you can truly and safely see and hear yourself and witness yourself, that awareness changes things. Suddenly the deception is over. So just your presence of care, compassion, safety, and trustworthiness as you enter the system, changes things.

But not always. If the kind of awareness you bring to yourself is judgmental awareness, you will make things worse. Then a downward negative spiraling begins. So that's where holding the frame in the context of *just exploring* to see what's there introduces non-judgmental awareness and pure witnessing. NLP got this idea of pure witnessing as a powerful change agent from Fritz Perls who said, "Lose your mind and come to your senses."

Third, there is the change factor of *changing the frame.* If the frame of meaning is the problem, then changing it, changes the person. Transformation occurs by altering the reference point. And whether it is an old belief, decision, understanding, prohibition, intention, identity, metaphor, etc., altering or reframing the mental map transforms things.

Two key change principles that we use in Neuro-Semantics are these.
>First, we can change no one, but as we change, the game changes and that invites others to change.
>Second, we can change no one, but we can facilitate another to choose to change.

Both of these principles empower you to give up the need to change people. Knowing that you can't, you then release others from the grip of your manipulations. And when you do, something magical happens. People change. They change because the pressure is off. And when the pressure is off, then the person is thrown back on one of the most important Neuro-Semantic principles: *The responsibility and freedom of choice point.*

Choice point can occur at any and every meta-level in a person's Matrix. By holding the frames, mirroring them back, providing a context of care and support, you invite a person to step back or step up and gain a larger or wider perspective. "Ah, this is what you have been thinking-feeling, believing, understanding, identifying with, etc., how is that?" It's an open-ended question and it is a question that begins to invite the person to a point of choice.

> "So what do you want to do? Do you like that belief? That prohibition? That intention? Does that understanding serve you well? Does that frame empower you as a person?"

These are quality control questions, because that's what they do. They invite the person to check the quality of their frames and at the same time they put the person at choice point. It is their life. What will they do? Perceiving at this higher level empowers them now with the *ability* to *respond* as so they choose. And this typically is creates a leverage for the changes that the person has been looking for.

Facilitating change in a person who has developed a strong enough sense of self (what we call ego-strength) moves through four stages: Motivation, Decision, Creation, and Integration. These are the four axes in the *Axes of Change Model* of Neuro-Semantics which was originally designed for the Meta-Coaching System. That is, to facilitate a person through the change process requires four resources:

*   *Energy or motivation* to move away from what does not work and energy to move toward one's dreams, visions, and hopes— the life that a person wants to experience. Is there enough energy in the person's mind-body system to invest the effort for change? If no, work the motivation axes. If yes, then move to the next resource.

*   *Decisiveness* to make an informed and clearly weighed decision for paying the price that the change will require. Has the person

weighed the pros and cons of making the change and of not making the change? Is the person crystal clear about the price that he or she will pay for making the decision for or against the change? If no, then probe the person's pros and cons and the values inherent in each and then challenge them to make the decision. If yes, then move on to the next resource.

- *A creative new vision* mapped out as a blueprint of the new life chosen and a plan for innovating this creativity in everyday life. With the preparation for change completed, now comes the research and development phase as the person puts together a plan or a strategy for the change. Does the person know with precision and clarity what and how she will make the change happen? Does the person have a time-table and schedule for beginning to innovate and actualize the plan? If no, then work the creation axes. If yes, then move on to the next resource.

- *An integration in life-style* so that the new change is now in muscle-memory as the person's way of being in the world. Change created and begun won't last if not practiced in a disciplined way until it becomes automatic and one's default program. Have you reinforced and celebrated that successful steps so that a person finds the effort rewarded and the pattern now integrated? Have you begun the continuous improvement of testing the pattern to see what else could be taken to a new level? If no, then work the integration axes. If yes, then what's the next change you want to embrace and experience?

Facilitating change in Neuro-Semantics can occur in that deliberate, conscious, and methodical way; it can also occur in a more unconscious and holistic way. For that we use *The Crucible Model*.[8] This model utilizes the key change ingredients of Carl Rogers (unconditional positive regard, accurate empathy, and authenticity) along with other ingredients from Maslow, May, etc.— witnessing, acceptance, responsibility, and appreciation. Put all these together into a metaphorical space that brings out a person's best and you can then create a crucible space where old learnings can be reprocessed and the heat of truth—response-ability—and appreciation can come together for a transformation. The clue that it works is an ecstasy of falling back in love with life, with self, with others, with meaningfulness.[8]

Premise 8: Neuro-Semantics facilitates an unleashing of potentials that enables the transformation of personality, identity, and life's purpose. Finally, all of these premises culminate in the premise of self-actualization. It was Maslow and Rogers who postulated that *the self-actualization drive* is our most fundamental drive of all. It is the drive to keep moving forward and upward in making real (actualizing) what is clamoring within you. This life-long and never-ending drive is a drive to be real, to *be* who and what you are, and to keep transcending and including your current life situation.

This is a drive for *becoming* increasingly more and more authentic so that you unleash your real self. And in doing that, then you step into "the zone" or the "flow" zone, or the "genius" state of experiencing and giving yourself to that which makes you come truly alive and make a contribution that makes a difference in the world.[9]

Here's a paradox: while self-actualization has the term "self" within it, *it is not about you.* It is about actualizing yourself— your gifts, abilities, potentials, etc. so that you can truly contribute what is uniquely yours to contribute. And in that way, you truly make a difference in the world.

Neuro-Semantic Learnings for a Neuro-Semanticist
Okay, so what have you learned? If there's anything that people usually take away from Neuro-Semantic trainings it is that *unless something is getting into muscle-memory and being embodied, it is not real and won't become real.* So to make it real, to make it last, two questions:

> 1) What have you learned? What will you take away with you from reading this chapter? What speaks to you and inspires you?

> 2) How will you integrate that learning and make it yours so that it begins to change things? Will you write about it? Reflect upon it? Speak about it to someone? Turn it into a statement that you can repeat and put into your own words? Will you use the Mind-to-Muscle Pattern and incorporate it in your neurology?

If you have been in the presence of learning something significant, then make a decision right now that you will not leave the scene of your learning without making a life-changing decision.

End of the Chapter Notes

1. See *User's Manual of the Brain, Volume I* for the basic NLP Communication model and for instructions about the process of anchoring.

2. See *Meta-States: Managing the Higher Levels of the Mind.* Other books on Meta-States include: *Winning the Inner Game, Secrets of Personal Mastery,* and *Meta-States Magic.*

3. See *Dragon Slaying.* This book uses the metaphor of a "dragon" as an unresourceful state that you can tame, transform, or slay. Contrary to what some people say, "slaying" a dragon does not harm an endangered species. It is just a metaphor. And the other two verbs indicate that we most often tame them or transform their energies.

4. Training in this quality of listening and supporting occurs at the NLP Practitioner level and is benchmarked and taken to the next level in the *Coaching Mastery* program, module III of Meta-Coaching.

5. The danger here is manipulation. And there have been, and are, many who are misusing this fundamental human power. That's why we emphasize respect, care, and love in Neuro-Semantics and have a code of ethics in how to use this technology.

6. See *Structure of Personality.* In this book we explore the personality disorders of the DSM IV and show how NLP and Neuro-Semantics provides processes for addressing these more serious problems.

7. See *NLP Going Meta* for a chapter on Alfred Korzybski's role in Neuro-Semantics. There is also a chapter on Gregory Bateson and Robert Dilts as well.

8. See *The Crucible.*

9. See *Accessing Personal Genius* training manual, or *Secrets of Personal Mastery* (1999).

Chapter 2

MEANING-MAKING

The Human Adventure

"Nothing means anything on its own. Meaning comes not from seeing or even observation alone, for there is no 'alone' in this sort. Neither is meaning lying around in nature waiting to be scooped up by the senses; rather it is *constructed*. 'Constructed' in this context means produced in acts of interpretation."
Humberto R. Maturana

"What an organism does is organize, and what a human organism organizes is meaning. It is not that a person makes meaning as much as that the activity of being a person is the activity of meaning-making. There is thus no feeling, no experience, no thought, no perception, independent of a meaning-making context in which it *becomes* a feeling, an experience, a thought, a perception, because we *are* the meaning-making context."
Robert Kegan, *The Evolving Self,* (p. 11)

I n Neuro-Semantics the art of making, constructing, inventing, and construing meaning is the human adventure par excellence. It is what we all do. This is inescapable and inevitable. It is an adventure because it is about discovery, learning, invention, evaluation, experimentation, refining, etc. In Neuro-Semantics, this is our primary focus.

Why is meaning-making the essence of the human adventure? Because by nature and birth, by genetics and neurology— we don't know what anything means. Innately, we don't know what anything is, what it does, how it works, what it leads to, its value and importance, or how to cope with it. In this we are without the kind of "instincts" that animals have. In the place of instincts, the unique human adventure is that of constructing our meanings and our sense of reality.

Unlike the animals who are born with *content knowledge* about their domain of life—what things are, how they work, how to handle or cope with things, *we are born instinct-less.* This does not mean that we are a blank slate at birth; we are not. We have predispositions, brains wired with certain strengths and weaknesses, and general tendencies to be actualized. Yet we only have a general impulse or urge within, which we call our "drives" or "needs," so this lack of content information about our urges drives us to find out what they are and how they work. Maslow described this by saying that we have *instinctoids*—"left-over remnants of instincts" which we experience as urges, impulses, drives, and needs.

So without proper instincts—we are clueless, innocent, naive, vulnerable, and completely open to learning. At birth we are completely open to learning because we do not know—*innately we know nothing!* So if we have any "instinct," it is the instinct to learn. In fact, I think we can safely say, *Learning is the primary human drive.* From the beginning we are driven to learn what things mean—what they are, how they work, what they lead to, how to handle them. And this is precisely what we see in the infant and young child— a passion to learn, to explore, to find out, to make sense of things. This drive is also our basic meaning-making drive for self-actualization.

This drive is obviously important because when you don't know what something is, how it works, what it leads to—you don't know what to do. Should you approach or avoid? Is it safe or dangerous? Is it eatable or poisonous? And observing a young infant or child at work in their business of discovery, when they encounter things in their world that they don't know, they are intensely curious to find out more about it. That's why we have to "kid proof" our homes so that the things they do get into are safe to play with and put in their mouths!

To respond effectively to the objects, events, happenings, and people in our environment, we have to have some knowledge of it. We have to make sense of it and have a basic understanding of it. This is the first dimension of meaning. And from there, many more follow:

- What is this? What do I call this? How do I classify this?
- What does it do? Does it do anything? How does it work? What can I use it for?
- What does it lead to? What results from using this? What consequences will occur from interacting with it?
- What do others think and understand about this? Does it have any inter-personal or social value? If so, what?
- How does one handle or cope with this? Are there ways of handling this that make it dangerous? What are the most effective ways to handle this?
- Why use this? What are the common intentions and purposes that people bring to interacting with this?

How Meaning Works

As you can see from this list of questions, *meaning and meaning-making throbs as the heart pulse at the core of your life.* You have to figure things out in order to be able to respond effectively. As such meaning refers to a whole range of concepts. Here is a fundamental list of concepts inherent in the idea of *meaning*:

- *Identity*— what *it is.*
- *Classifications* — categories of understanding.
- *Conceptual understanding* —how it works.
- *Causation and correlation* —what it causes or leads to.
- *Coping, interacting, dealing with things* —what to do about it.
- *Intention* —purpose in dealing with it.
- *Values* —what is its significance or importance.
- *Source* —where does it come from.
- *Metaphor* —what is it like; what can it be compared to.
- *Story* —what narrative form can it take.

So when we speak about "the search for meaning," we are seeking to figure out any one, or all, of these things. *Meaning-making* is a phrase for how you make your mental models or maps about things— about the world you live in, the life you have, the relationships you are embedded in, what you can do, etc. So, how does meaning work? Or rather, how do you construct your mental models by which you make sense of the world? To answer that, let me tell you a story.

In the Beginning

It all begins with an experience.   If you do not come loaded with meaning constructs ("instincts"), and if you have to "make" sense of things by constructing mental models, then it begins with the encounters and experiences you have with the world. As you *sense* the world with your senses—you begin to experience what is "out there" in the world.

Psychologically, this is the first level of meaning-making, *the unspeakable level* that activates and engages your body and neurology. Here you make connections and associations so that your most primitive level of consciousness is that of being a sensate and sentient being—*aware of the world and taking cognizance of it.* At this level, which occurs from birth to about nine months, your undeveloped brain does not and cannot make and hold internal representations of the world which is why "out of sight is out of mind" for the infant.

Developmental psychologists call the ability to bring in the outside world "constancy of representation." You are now able to bring the outside world inside your mind via what you see and hear on the outside and re-present inside, in your mind—your mental constructs. Prior to nine months, you are not able to do this. That's why the game of bee-a-boo works so delightfully with infants. We put something between us and the baby and suddenly pop out from behind the barrier and, surprise of surprise!   "You are there! Where did you come from!" The baby is surprised, delighted, giggling. The child experiences a cognitive jar.[1]

Until that age the baby also stops exploring for something when he can no longer see something. After that age, however, the baby will continue to pursue an object or a face and use his or her hands to try to remove the barrier.   Apparently the baby now has sufficient "constancy of representation" to know that the object is still there, just hidden from sight.

And with this new power of representing
something and holding it in mind, something
truly fabulous, wonderful, incredible, even
"magical" happens—*we bring inside
ourselves the things that occur outside.* We represent the world of sights,
sounds, sensations, smells, tastes, and words. We can hold "the world" that
we experience on the outside inside our mind! We hold in mind what we
have experienced via our senses on the outside. And "holding" something
in mind is what the word *meaning* means (e.g., "to hold in mind"). Now, as
it were, you can take the world with you. Prior to this, mom and dad's night
out was an utter terror. But now you can hold "mom and dad" in mind, on
the theater of your mind and comfort yourself by doing so.

> The word *meaning* means
> "to hold in mind."

Cognitive Stages of Making Meaning

The first level of meaning is actually before awareness, the *unspeakable level*
whereby the energies in the world "out there" impact your senses and
neurology. The problem here, of course, is that you lack awareness of this
level. It occurs without your awareness—your neurology receives it and is
"aware" of it, but you are not.

After that comes the representational level. And at first, this also is outside-
of-consciousness. You may be representing something in your "mind," but
lack awareness of that awareness. And yet your visual, auditory, associative
cortexes are working so that you are developing meanings about what is out
there and your experiences with those things and activities. Your cognitive
unconscious is processing information.

At this level of your "mind," you are noticing the world—seeing, hearing,
smelling, sensing, tasting, etc. and yet without awareness of doing so. You
are sensitive to your environment, taking it in, processing the datum that is
before you.

Next comes the level wherein *you become aware of your representations.*

As the brain develops during childhood, children move into the concrete thinking stage (7 to 11 years) wherein they confuse their thoughts with what's real. If they think it, it must be real. For them, the map *is* the territory. That's what makes them such absolutists! This also is what can make their inner life so terrifying because if they think they see a monster in the closet, there *is* a monster in the closet! And our denials do not reassure them. They take their thoughts as real and absolute. The meanings they make are absolute and real (to them).

Children at this stage are ego-centric in that they see the world through their absolutist maps of the world. They are not yet able to step out of their thinking and take another person's perspective.

Stages of Cognitive Development	
Years	*Stage*
0 to 2	*Sensiormotor* Schemes through senses and motor activities
2 to 7	*Pre-operational* Acquisition of ability to conserve and decenter
7 to 11	*Concrete operational* Capable of operations (reversibility)
11 to 14	*Formal operational* Able to generalize to hypothetical experiences, deal with abstractions, form hypothesis

So when they play "Hide and Seek," they may stand still, close their eyes, and because they can't see their playmates, they assume that no one can see them. If they see someone hide something in a drawer when another friend is not in the room, when asked if the friend knows where it is, they say, "Of course." They know, and they can't imagine that everyone would not know.

At the end of the concrete operational stage (11 to 14 years), as the brain keeps developing, one's concreteness loosens up. Now the child begins to become free from the concreteness in which he or she has been embedded and free for a wider and more expansive meaning-making sense. At this stage they begin to realize that their view of the world is not absolute, that others operate according to their own mental models. Now they can begin to realize that their thinking is *their* thinking and everyone doesn't see, perceive, understand, believe, or think the same as they do. This introduces the "time of secrets." They now discover that they can keep secrets from the big people, that mom and dad cannot really read their minds. They have a private place! They may test this for awhile by lying.[2]

The final cognitive stage, formal abstract thinking, comes with puberty, when there is the maturity of the physical brain and the release of hormones that completes the development of the brain. Now the young adult can truly step aside from his or her thinking and create abstract meanings about things.

Figure 2:1

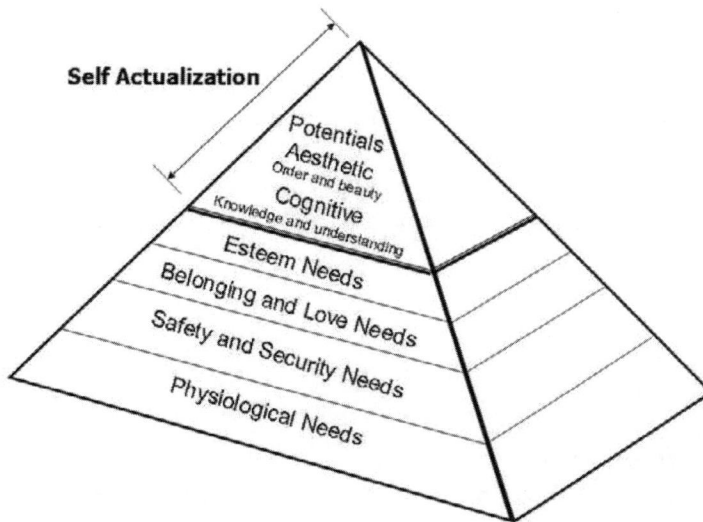

Self Actualization

Potentials
Aesthetic
Order and beauty
Cognitive
Knowledge and understanding
Esteem Needs
Belonging and Love Needs
Safety and Security Needs
Physiological Needs

Cognitive Coping

At the same time that you are first making meaning with your primitive brain as an infant and slowly growing through the stages of cognitive development, your basic instinctoids are creating *impulses that are energizing you* to figure out *what* they are and *how* to cope with them. No wonder the infant and child could not survive without a nurturing community—caretakers who already understand and know *what* the child needs, *what* impulses and needs are driving the developing person, and *how* to cope with those drives effectively.

It is much later that you begin to cognitively find out about these basic needs and come to understand them and figure out how to cope with them. So even before you are ready or able to create *meanings* that will be accurate, useful, and practical, you are thrown into the human dilemma of feeling and experiencing your needs and trying to figure them out.

> "What are these impulses? Is this hunger, fear, excitement, wonder, play, etc.? What should I do to quiet these inner urges?"

At this point in my description, two models of human development emerge—Maslow's Hierarchy of Needs and Piaget's Cognitive Development stages. The first things you need to create *meaning* about are your internal needs and your external life context. This enables you to move through the Hierarchy of Needs from all of your survival needs, then safety needs, then social (love and affection) needs, and your self needs. While we will return to this in chapter 9, here is a brief overview of the hierarchy of needs.[3]

Survival Needs:

> What is happening? Is this thing, person, animal, and event something that supports my life or does it threaten life? First you try to make sense of the various aspects of survival—air, water, food, sleep, health, money, etc.

Safety Needs:

> Is this person or thing safe or dangerous? Is it friend or foe? Is this

good for me, neutral, or poisonous? Will this create stability and order in my life or chaos and confusion? Can I be safe enough to relax, to learn, and to explore? Do I have some control in life?

Social Needs:

Is this person nurturing and caring or hurtful and dangerous? Can this person provide love and affection for me? Are my needs important or unimportant to this person? Will I feel connected, bonded, close, and loved?

Self Needs:

Do I count? Am I important? Do I have any value as a person? What can I do that is unique and special with me? Where do I stand in the community of people that I live among? Do they believe in me or not?

These needs, which you experience as inner impulses driving you to gratify them, are governed by the principle of *deficiency*. You experience them when you need them, when you lack them, when you have a deficiency of the things that would gratify that need. The more deficiency, the greater the intensity of the impulse and urge. In fact, as the deficiency grows in intensity, you can become absolutely desperate. And that is when you are likely to do desperate things that can hurt yourself and others. And yet when the needs are truly gratified, the urge and impulse simply goes away. And you then typically experience a post-gratification forgetting—forgetting how driving they were and how desperate you felt.

Stimulus—Response Meaning-Making

At first in your meaning-making, you use pain/pleasure as your sole criteria for making distinctions. "This hurts." "That feels good." Pain / pleasure, comfort/discomfort, struggle/ease therefore establish your first epistemology for "good" and "bad." During childhood, you mostly make meanings through associations and connections. This creates your *associative meanings*. So meaning at this level operates as strictly a Stimulus—Response (S-R) interaction and construction:

"When stimulus X occurs, I respond in Y or Z way Y or Z thoughts, feelings, and reactions."

Meaning in this format is simple association or linkage. You link one event to another simply because they occurred about the same time. One child creates the meaning: "Picking up a book of matches is associated with being spanked, equals pain." Another child creates another meaning: "Picking up a book of matches means getting mom's disapproval, equals I feel unloved." Yet another invents the meaning: "Picking up a book of matches is a lot of fun, but must be done privately away from the prying eyes of parents."

Stimulus followed by a response may be a mere correlation or accident and not necessarily a cause, yet you may "make sense" of the relationship between events by thinking of it as a "cause." The meaning you make is that "This stimulus causes that response." "When event X happens, it makes me feel or respond in Y." Structurally, this is a stimulus—response meaning (S—>R). "Loud sound scares me." "Rubbing my tummy, and saying soothing words makes me feel better."

The associative meaning-making of this kind of neuro-semantic experience is simple in structure and creates your first thinking and believing structures. "X causes Y." In this way you create your first mental-emotional mappings about the world. It is the best you can do with the primitive and under-developed brain that you have at that time. Later your meaning-making will become more sophisticated and complex as you realize that the world cannot be so simply explained.

In terms of your personal meaning-making history, you begin your mental modeling of the world with these simplistic linear cause-effect meanings. Later these generalizations become your beliefs about yourself, others, and the world at large. At first this helps you to organize the chaotic confusion of the world as you give it some order and structure. Obviously, you have to begin somewhere and developmentally, this is where we all begin.

> "Harsh tonalities make me feel bad. I'm going to get hurt."
> "Not knowing something makes me embarrassed. People in authority (teachers, parents) hate me when I don't know something."
> "To make a mistake is to risk punishment. It is bad and painful to make mistakes."[4]

Figure 2:2

S—>R

Stimulus — Response

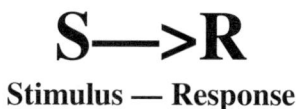

External Behavior —> Internal State
Events in the World —> Internal Experiencing
See, Hear, Feel, etc. Stimuli —> Thinking, Feeling

Referential Thinking — *What are You Referring to?*

As your thinking begins with sensory-perception, it quickly becomes association or reference. *Your experiences make up the stuff you use as your references for making meaning.* If you could carry on a conversation at that stage and ask, "What does a strained voice mean?" and a child says, "I'm bad, in danger, or terribly afraid." We could then ask, "What are you referring to that gives you these ideas and these feelings?" Their thinking and meaning-making comes from some experience and that experience is their *reference* for how they have come to that conclusion.

Your meaning-making begins most fundamentally by using *some reference for how you reason, interpret, and construe the world.* Ultimately all of us use our sensory experiences of seeing, hearing, smelling, feeling, and tasting as our first point of reference. To create meaning you cannot select every experience, so you first have to select some experience. So as you choose to focus on some event, you select that event to reason from. How you construe that event, the thinking patterns you use to interpret it, then governs the meanings that you create from it.

This description identifies how we think by referring to some event or situation (referencing). When you think or have a thought, you first have to have *a thought about something.* Once you think and select it, you represent it inside, and from there you begin to "make sense" of it by classifying it, labeling it, evaluating it, interpreting it, etc. You "reason" about it. You draw conclusions.

The meaning-making process not only starts with some reference, it continues using references. As you draw a conclusion, that *conclusion now becomes what you are referring to when you conceptually move up to the next level of awareness.* The only difference is that you move from an external reference (the original event or experience) to internal references as your mental structures.   And at first, you will not even be aware that you are dong this. In this sense, all of your higher mental functions are just the references or contexts that you have created. So to understand yourself or another person, we ask about the references a person is using as he or she constructs a Matrix of frames about that something.[5]

Representational Thinking as First-Level Reference
You begin your meaning-making by bringing the world inside yourself as you represent an experience—the one you refer to when you think about learning, playing, taking a test, making a mistake, etc. Then using your brain neurology, you *present-to-yourself-again* (re-present) that external referent. We call this experience "thinking" and name this process with the noun-like word, "mind."   And then we treat the mind *as if* it were a movie theater where you see and hear and even feel the experience. What you *see* externally, you can *see* again on the inside as you *re*call and *re*cognize the referent. All of this is still a mystery in the neuro-sciences. What I'm describing is not a literal description, that's why it is an *as if* seeing. The first *seeing* you did with your eyes as you used them as sense receptors, the second *seeing* is as you *re*member and use it as your next level reference. Literally, there are no pictures in your mind, or sounds, it just *seems* that way as you make meaning.

You also do this with all of your senses. What you *hear* on the outside, you now *hear* again on the inside by recalling and rehearsing. Again, we call this "thinking" or self-talk. It is meaning-making because you are holding in mind what you brought in from the outside. What you *smell, taste,* and *sense* (feel) externally, you now smell, taste, and feel on the inside. It takes a more developed mind to engage in such internal rehearsal as you represent the original referent and use it as your reference. At first you do all of this without being conscious of these functions, eventually however you begin to become aware of what's occurring within your mind. And when you do that you can begin to take charge of these processes.

Apparently cats and dogs and other higher forms of mammals engages in this process. They can *recognize* (*re-* "again;" *cognize*, "think") people, places, things, events, commands, etc. But as far as we can tell, they lack awareness that they are doing this. They just do it. They are sentient, but they are not aware of their sentience. The higher parts of their cortex enable them to do it as the higher parts of our cortex also allows us to do it. Yet they are not self-aware as you and I are.

The *referencing* skills lead to higher and higher levels of thinking. Animals use *signals* to refer to things. The barking, jumping, rolling over, purring, etc., as part of an experience, refers to the experience. The growl, as part of the attack, refers to imminent or possible danger. We humans, however, use full fledged *symbols*, that is, we can and do use arbitrary sounds, images, movements, etc. to stand for something other than itself.[6]

This level of development of referencing starts with *pointing*. Parents point to the things they are referring to and give them names and labels. "Daddy," "Mommy," "spoon," "brother," "table," "food."

I once pointed to a window and said to my cat, "Window, go." My cat just looked at my finger. Then he gingerly licked it, turned up his nose, and went back to sleep. "Not interested," I deduced. His attitude seemed to be, "If the pointing finger isn't good for licking or eating, what good is it? It's irrelevant." It stood for itself. It pointed to nothing. "Pointing" as an activity of referencing, as symbol that stood for something else, "Look there!" meant nothing to my cat, Ferocious.

In meaning-making we begin with references that we can point to—they are point-able. You can *use your finger* by pointing your finger to the object. The world of *finger-able things* is the world of sensory-based things and processes. We use nouns and verbs to point these things out: house, car, desk, coat, shoes, etc.

Figure 2:3

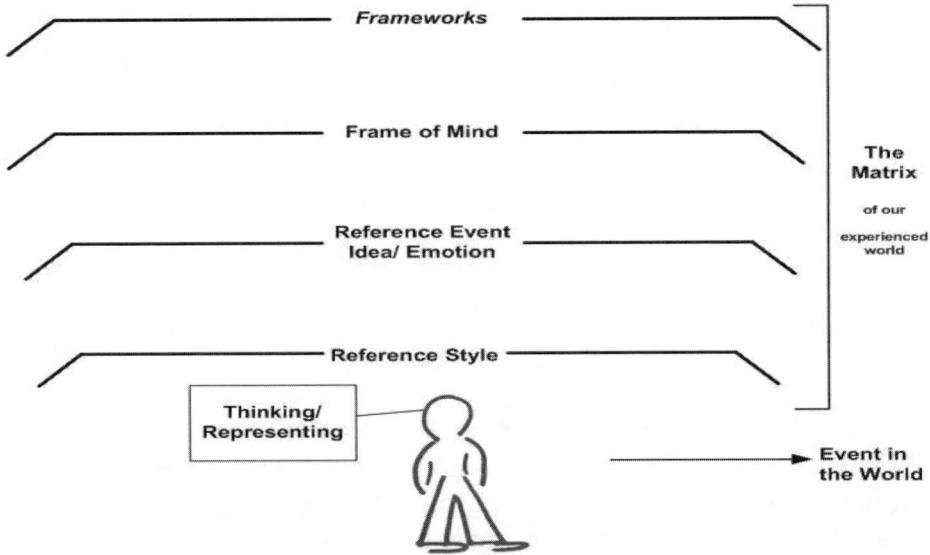

Then there are lots of things in our mental-emotional world that are not finger-able, they are *un-finger-able*: justice, relationship, communication, meaning, dignity, power, responsibility, honor, love, faith, intention, etc. In fact, come to think of it—the things that matter most to us are all un-finger-able. You can't put your finger on them. When you point to them, you are figuratively pointing to a concept of your mind.

So when you ask referencing questions about things not seen, heard, or felt in the sensory-based world, you have moved to a higher level of mind, and to references that are in *mental frames-of-reference.*
> "What do you mean by that concept?"
> "What understanding, belief, value, etc. are you referring to?"

In the process of meaning-making you move to the next level when you mentally refer to experiences, events, people, ideas, etc.—experiences beyond the scope of see-hear-feel world. In doing this you transcend that world and enter into a higher world— *a world of mind, communication, meaning, and information* (Bateson's terminology). Here you "understand" things, create concepts, develop beliefs, and give meaning to things. Here you associate or link up levels of meanings (meanings about meanings).

> What does justice mean to you? What do you believe about human nature?
>
> What do you refer to when you talk about beauty or goodness?

Frame / Framing

An interpretive scheme, a way to structure consciousness and information. From "frame of reference" the internal context held in mind as a lens.

So in building up layers of references you create *layers of meanings* about things. What began as an external reference, becomes a represented reference, then an evaluated frame of reference, then a frame of mind, etc.

External Referent Becomes Internal

Let's say that you perceive and notice that your dad gets upset with you make a mistake and raises his voice at you. He yells at you. As he does so, the tension in his body, especially in his neck, causes his voice to have a harsh tone. As dad yells, child feels bad. Perhaps even scared. Perhaps the child construes this situation as disappointed with himself. Perhaps he interprets it as being disappointed with dad. Perhaps he feels ashamed of being caught at doing something wrong.

Let's suppose this happens repeatedly, or at least every once in a while. Now the child begins to anticipate it. He creates an internal representation of his dad getting upset, looking tense, stressed, and speaking in a strained voice. Now within the child's mental world, and on the theater of his mind (consciously or unconsciously), he has *a represented reference* as a mental model or a template that he uses to explain the event and to which he then responds.

Suppose further that even before the child makes a mistake, he uses this representation as his reference for what to expect. Doing this moves the child up a level—he has layered these thoughts and emotions. His representation is now an internal frame of reference. He now sees his dad and other experiences through the lens of this previous experience. His meaning-making of this "memory," that is, his *expectations,* now colors his world.

Now "harsh tonality" and a "stern face" is no longer a mere perception to notice and inquire about. Now it is a template, or frame, for processing information, i.e., taking a chance, making a mistake, encountering dad, etc. In this way the representations are elaborated into a layered and complex understanding that operates as a self-fulfilling prophesy.

This move in meaning-making moves the child to a higher level as *he sets a frame about his representations.* From now on, with his understanding about harsh tones, whenever he hears a harsh tonality, he has a reference or an internal context for understanding it. *He has framed it.* He processes it by using his mental construction. And yes, this saves time and trouble as he does not have to start afresh in trying to understand what it is, what it means, what to do. But on the other side, he loses sensory awareness and the ability to be in the here-and-now without pre-judgments:

> "Harsh tonalities make me feel bad."
> "Harsh tonalities mean I'm going to get hurt."
> "It's bad to speak with a harsh tonality."

What was originally at the content level of information about a specific incident has now moved to become a frame—*a frame of reference for interpreting things.* This creates a first level frame of reference. Later if the boy begins to believe it, he sets it as part of his interpretative style. By the way, with that frame, he has the structure for a *frame game.* His frames, as his inner game enables him to play outer games: *It's a Big, Bad, Terrifying World Out There. Bad Tonality Makes You a Bad Person.* The rules that govern this game enables him to have ready access to feeling terrified, threatened, violated, and abused whenever someone speaks with that tone of voice.[7]

In the inner landscape of the boy's mind, he now has a frame— a frame of reference— that he uses to "understand" his world, to "know" what's going on, to feel, and to respond. He has created "meaning."

Linguistic Meaning-Making
As you and I construct meanings from associations, representations, and stimulus-response linkages, we use words. We use words to label things. You classify the events, things, and people that you encounter and I classify

things as I encounter them. You categorize using various linguistic terms and descriptions, so do I. So at the primary level of meaning-making, we not only use sensory-based representations and thus the representational systems, we also use words.

At first words are the labels that we put upon things and people—so we use nouns. Then we begin using words that describe actions and processes—this gives us verbs. After that we begin using words that hold sentences together and that give them a particular linguistic structure. Eventually, our words become more and more abstract so that they lose their direct relationship to the sensory representational systems. And as this happens, you shift more and more of your thinking and meaning-making to language so that your words become your linguistic tools for constructing meaning.

The challenge linguistic meaning offers is that language is several steps removed from the experience at the unspeakable level. It has been transformed by neurology into the "senses" that you can detect, then it has been selected, filtered, foregrounded, backgrounded, and represented in your unique way, then finally we get to sensory-based *descriptive words*. After that through more transformations, abstractions, and interpretations, the words become increasingly evaluative and can become completely disconnected to the original experience.

Appreciating How You Create Meaning

By way of summary, you at first *link* and *associate* to reduce the amount of confusion and chaos in the world. You construct your first mappings of what things mean in this way.

> *"What does something mean?"*

It depends what you or another person has connected to a thing, event, or word. How do they represent it and, given that representation, what is that linked to? "Meaning" does not have to be logical, rational, or valid in this sense. That's why *associative meaning* can be so idiosyncratic and unique to a given individual and that without understanding the historical context within which the person linked up the connections, we have a difficult time understanding the person's "logic."

In *Mind-Lines: Lines for Changing Minds* (1998/ 2005),[4] I found the following story and included it as an example of associative meaning:

"In one of the big earthquakes that shook southern California in the 1980s—just prior to the quake, a mother became upset with her little 5 year old for slamming a door in the house. Just as she began a new rebuke stating that "something really bad will happen if you keep doing this," the little boy slammed the door and then the whole house shook and trembled, dishes crashed to the floor, lamps came tumbling down, etc. This absolutely terrified the little boy —who *in his nervous system*—connected "slamming the door" with causing an Earthquake. He also connected, "arguing with mom" as leading to an earthquake." (p. 201)

A very special kind of *logic* arises inside the human nervous system when you associate or link one thing with another. This linkage does not have to fit the criteria for "logical" in any formal sense. It is the "logic" of association. It "makes sense" of the world in terms of simple association or linkage.

"This X happened (sassing mom, talking back) and then this Y happened (earthquake, house devastated, emotional state of intense fear, even terror). So the X must have caused the Y. Speaking up to mom is really dangerous, threatening, terror producing."

This kind of thinking in a five-year-old in response to those events probably reflects the best thinking for a child of that age. Most twenty-year-old minds would not have created that map. An adult mind would have mapped it out with a fuller and more mature understanding, being able to apply other frames-of-references to the situation: knowledge of earthquakes, the ability to separate events that occur sequentially or simultaneously in terms of the concept of "causation," etc. Again, this is the "logic" that Korzybski referred to when he put a hyphen in psychology, to create the term, *psycho-logics.*

As the child so maps it out, so he thinks, knows, and feels. It becomes "real" inside the person's body. His very neurology experiences it as "real." The linguistics that he maps out in his mind, "sassing mom makes bad things happen," creates powerful neurological effects throughout his entire body, brain, physiology, and nervous system. It has induced what we call a *neuro-linguistic state of consciousness.*

You and I do the same thing using our own unique expereinces. You have this wonderful, magical, and powerful ability to connect all kinds of irrational things together and to then *feel* that it is *absolutely real and unquestionable.* All of your "intuitions" confirm it! Just try to convince someone otherwise.

> "Silly you, I *know* better! The way my heart and lungs beat when I think about misbehaving, slamming a door, speaking up to an authority figure, etc., what craziness to suggest that it could be otherwise!"

Once you link one thing with another thing, your brain, nervous system, and all of your connecting human tissue "knows," at a neurological level, that "sassing mom creates devastating effects!" This creates one of the things that we mean by "intuitions," or "intuitive" knowledge. It illustrates a fact that I'll describe later in chapter 9: "The meaning you give is the instinct you will live.*"

It's Frames of Reference all the Way Up
This describes the beginning of the human adventure of meaning-making. There's more and I'll describe more of that adventure in the next chapter in the *Levels of Meaning.*

Neuro-Semantic Learnings for a Neuro-Semanticist
Now you know about the human adventure of creating meaning. You know that it is the adventure that arises because you are free to invent and discover meanings. Meaning is not given in your genetics or neurology— you get to be your own creator of meanings. And the adventure takes a lifetime. Given all of this what are you taking away from this chapter? What have you learned about the meaning-making processes?

> 1) How will this information about meaning-making influence you as a meaning-maker? How conscious are you of your internal representations? How much control would you gauge that you have over those representations?

2) If meaning always goes back to some referent event, experience, or words, and if it's a matter of selection — that is, you could have selected other facets of the experience to focus on, what changes will you make about the references you have been using to build your meanings on?

End of Chapter Notes

1. See the work of Eric Erickson, Jean Piaget, Robert Kegan, Fowler.

2. Paul Tournier, *Secrets* (1963).

3. See Maslow's classic work on the hierarch, *Motivation and Personality* (1954/ 1970). Also *Self-Actualization Psychology* (2009) and *Unleashed* (2007).

4. This is fully developed in the book, *Mind-Lines: Lines for Changing Minds* (2005) and more fully utilized in chapter 14.

5. "Matrix" literally means "a womb," and designates a place where something is given birth. In Neuro-Semantics we use it as a metaphor of your internal sets of meanings where you give birth to all of your ideas. This has led to the Matrix Model (2003) as a systems model for working with meaning and consciousness.

6. See Gregory Bateson, *Steps to an Ecology of Mind* (1972).

7. This introduces the word *frame* as we use it in Neuro-Semantics which goes back to the work of Gregory Bateson.

Chapter 3

THE KINDS

OF MEANING

"Experience is not what happens to you,
it is what you *do* with what happens to you."
Aldous Huxley, 1972

"Man is in the business to make sense of the world
and to test the sense he has made in terms of its predictive capacity."
Don Bannister and Fay Fransella

When it comes to the meanings that you and I, as meaning-makers, make—there are many questions. Here we will be exploring the *kinds, levels,* and *dimensions* of meaning. Afterwards we will explore the *quality* and *ecology* of the meanings. This is essential because before you can actualize your highest and best, you first have to find and create inspiring meanings for your life—meanings that are wonderful, exciting, and that elicit your highest visions and passions. You can't unleash your potential without creating great meanings which unleash your energies.

This chapter focuses first on a critical aspect of meaning and meaning-making—*the kinds* of meanings that you make, *the levels* at which you construct these meanings, and the various *dimensions* of meaning.

Kinds of Meanings

The mystery of meaning, as what you "hold in mind," is that meaning can have many different expressions. And given that there's all kinds of meanings, *all meanings are not the same.* There are associative meanings and representational meanings. There are framed meanings and belief meanings. And there's more— there's a *lot* more! Here is an enumerated list of some of the most basic kinds of meanings that we all deal with and that govern the content of our consciousness.

1) *Associative meaning*

The first meanings that you make are the associative meanings that happen by accident— accident of time, space, birth, environment, context. That is, you come to invent, make, and construct "meaning" out of whatever is nearby when you link and associate with another thing. If, as an infant you see or hear or touch something and the next response is one of comfort, pleasure, delight, and fun—you will likely connect a "good" association with that item. The experience is reinforced. If the next thing that happens is unpleasant, painful, distressful, that's what gets connected.

2) *Evaluative meaning*

Once you associate one thing with another, then you make some evaluation about it. Is it good for you or not? Does it promote your well-being or undermine your well-being? Do you like it or hate it? To evaluate something is to view it through the lens of your values or criteria. "In terms of this experience being fun—it is or it is not fun." So this kind of meaning arises from the development of standards. Every standard, everything that you decide is important to you (a value) then becomes a means by which you make an evaluation or judgment.

3) *Metaphorical meaning*

Metaphor represents another kind of meaning. This is the meaning that you construct when you compare one thing to another thing. "I felt like I had a tiger by the tail." "As I stood up there on stage, I felt like a car wreck was about to happen." In metaphorical meaning, you speak about one thing but you reference another. It is meaning-by-analogy. "This X is like Y."

Of course, all words and all meaning are metaphorical in that we are creating a code about something in terms of something else. This is what it means to use symbols and, as a symbol-user, all languages are metaphorical and symbolic. You are always using some symbol or metaphor to speak about something else. "The map is not the territory."

Metaphorical meaning presents two particular dangers. The first danger is that you over-use it and, through habituation of the metaphor, eventually forget that it's a metaphor so that you take it literally. So while all language is metaphorical, most of the original metaphors have been lost in history so that the words we now use no longer seem metaphorical. Those that are in that process are considered cliches—over-used statements. In these the metaphor is no longer fresh.

The second danger is the connotations that come along with metaphors, what George Lakoff and Mark Johnson call "entailments" in Cognitive Linguistics. *An entailment* refers to all of the things that come along with the metaphor that does not fit the analogy. This explains why you can take and extend any and every metaphor too far, beyond what the metaphor can be applied to usefully, and create distortions.

As an example, the idea that there's an "inner child" within a person may be a useful metaphor to help complete some emotional or psychological business that feels not completed. But it's a metaphor. There is no literal child inside! Freud made use of the hydralic metaphor when he described emotions and how they need some way to release the steam as if they are blocked off, they will find some other way to get out. Well, the idea of emotions as energy is one thing, as steam energy seeking release, that's another thing and in my point of view, not a very useful or healthy one. I think it misunderstands the nature of how emoting occurs in our mind-body system (see chapter five).

4) *Representative Meaning*
The ideas that you hold in your mind by representing them on the screen of your mind (a metaphor) is representational meaning. This was the genius that Bandler and Grinder mapped out in great detail that launched NLP originally and that caught the appreciative critical mind of Gregory Bateson

as he indicated in his Preface to *The Structure of Magic*. Representational meaning using the sensory representational systems of visual, auditory, and kinesthetic provides us ways to manage and control our thinking and the states our cognitions evoke in us.

5) *Editorial Meaning*

In NLP the distinctions within each of the representational systems that indicate the qualities of the sights, sounds, sensations etc., originally called "pragma-graphics" and later changed to "sub-modalities," is another form of meaning.[1] It is the meaning of your how you *editorially frame or code your representations.* That is, with any inner mental movie, you can edit it as close or far, bright or dim, in color or black-and-white, big or small, etc. These qualities that you then give the representations gives them a certain feel or tone— it sets a certain frame about it.

I call them *editorial meanings,* rather than sub-modalities, because they are not smaller pieces of the movie, but meta-level or meta-modalities *about* the movie. To see any mental movie and to notice or change its features, you have to step back ("go meta" to it) and notice its structure. You are at the editorial level of consciousness *about* the movie. Now you can add color, remove color, bring it closer, move it farther away, add some circus music, do all kinds of things— just like an editor of a movie can re-code it and give it a new feeling and tone. So these *cinematic features* of the movie are not "sub" to it, but meta to it.

6) *Linguistic Meaning*

Another kind and form of meaning is that which shows up linguistically, in language. In fact, this is what we most commonly refer to as "meaning"— words, grammar, language. Yet it is obviously just one kind of meaning. Within a person's mental inner movie, there are words being said and recorded and then there are words that label and classify the movie. So language can operate at multiple levels and therefore function in different ways. Language *about* things performs the function of classifying, categorizing, and framing. And language itself can be used for so many different things—description, evaluation, connecting, disconnecting, blessing, cursing, de-stressing, asking, inquiring, asserting, imploring, bonding, committing, vowing, releasing, understanding, and so on.

The meaning of language covers these and many other functions. The myth about language is that most of our communications are non-verbal rather than verbal. But the old "7, 38, 55" is just that— *a myth.* And it is a myth that Dr. C. E. "Buzz" Johnson has exposed in his article, *The 7, 38, 55 Myth.*[2] The shocking expose that Dr. Johnson discovered was that those statistics were not even about human communication. They are about dog communication! And worse, they are about one-word utterances and how much of those one word utterances were understood/ communicated by words (7 percent), tone and volume and auditory qualities (38 percent), and visual facial and body expressions (55 percent). No wonder this does *not* fit human communciations!

With just your non-verbals, your tones and visual expressions, try to say, "Dinner will be at 6 p.m sharp, please be present." And you can not cheat by using sign language—that's a symbolic or language system. Or watch a movie in a language that you do not understand. Then watch it translated so you can understand it. How much did you pick up just seeing and hearing? How much did you pick up when you heard words you understood?

In terms of language, some of the most fundamental ways that linguistic "meaning" shows up are as follows:[3]
*   *Identification:* What is this or that thing? These are coded as names, labels, nominalizations, identifications (using the "to be" verb: is, am, are, was, were, be, being).
*   *Operations:* How does this or that thing work? This is coded as cause-effect (C-E) or as Mind-Reading (MR) statements.
*   *Significance:* What is its value? These will be coded as complex equivalences (CEq. This X = Y) and as nominalizations.
*   *Intention:* What is this thing's purpose, agenda, motivation, or intention?

7) *Perceptual Meaning*
When it comes to perceptual meaning, this is the making of meaning that results in your perceptual lens that governs what and how you see or perceive things from your point of view. It is your thinking patterns and your thinking style. Do you think optimistically or pessimistically? Which

ever style characterizes you, you have constructed meaning to such a degree that now the meaning has stuck and become so habituated, you see the world through those meanings. Those meanings are now your perceptual lens or which in NLP we call "meta-programs."[4]

With perceptual meaning, it seems that the meaning of something is "out there." That's how you see it. It looks optimistic or pessimistic, but it is not. "Out there" is just a glass that has water in it at a certain level. But you see and perceive it in a certain way. The meaning that governs your perception originally came from how you meta-stated it. That is, a meta-program is a solidified and integrated meta-state.[5]

8) *Intentional Meaning*
Sometimes we use the word meaning as a synonym of intention. When you ask, "What do you mean by doing that?" you are asking for the person's intention or purpose. "What I meant by that was X" you might say as you try to express the intention behind the communication that was misread. This kind of meaning comes from your intentional level of processing information.

All of these are different ways for encoding meaning. You can now use them as a checklist when you are exploring your own or another person's meanings about something. There are more of these kinds of meanings, yet with these, you have those that are the most important for your explorations (see Figure 3:1).

Layering of the Kinds of Meaning
As a meaning-maker who creates your reality by your meanings, *you also create meaning in levels* (chapter four). Instead of "instincts" you have within you a gap of knowing—it is within this gap that you learn and invent the meanings that you then live by. So if meaning is constructed, and if you construct it by *how* and *what* you think, then you call the structures, forms, energies, and meanings of your reality into existence.

Meaning is layered because whatever meaning you create about something, what you then reflectively think or feel *about* that becomes the meanings that you frame them in and which then become your internal context for understanding and interpretation. How will you layer level-upon-level of meanings to create your reality? What are the layers involved in the levels of meaning and the meta-questions that can enable us to construct a whole matrix of meaning?

Given these different kinds of meanings, and the fact of your self-reflexive consciousness, it is inevitable that you will generate layer upon layer of these different kinds of meanings as you "think" and "feel." Doing so generates your overall Matrix of frames of meaning about any facet of your life.

That meaning comes in levels or layers explains the "logical levels" (chapter four). Every time you classify something into a category, you create another "logical level." Every time you step back from your thinking-and-feeling experience, you access yet another level of thinking-and-feeling and so move up a level. Every time you transcend one awareness and include it in a larger perspective, you create another logical level.

These two nominalizations ("logical" and "level") describes the reflexivity process. It identifies how you transcend and include your thoughts-and-feelings into higher thoughts-and-feelings. Of course, literally there is no such "thing" as a "logical level." A "logical level" is not a thing at all, it is a process. It is process of layering these levels ("levels") of your reasoning ("logics").

And in terms of the meaning-making that you and I create with these "levels" of thoughts-and-feelings, there are an infinite amount of levels. Linguistically, we have identified over one hundred terms in Neuro-Semantics. And yet, here is a paradox—they all refer to the same thing, the some experience. A better metaphor is that of *the diamond of consciousness* (see end of chapter four). In this metaphor, each "level" is simply another *facet* of the diamond, another perspective, or avenue.

Climbing the Ladder of Meaning
Let's play with the metaphor of levels or layers. Doing so allows you to think of exploring, detecting, and understanding the layers of meanings as *climbing a ladder*—as moving up level after level to see how you or another has put together his or her psycho-logical levels.

Doing this enables you to begin to identify a person's sequence and structure of meaning. Yet these levels are not like solid steps. They are dynamic and so change and move as you enter to explore a human system. It's like the moving staircase in the Harry Potter movies. Further, after the first steps, there is no particular order for how to do this. Begin with the lower distinctions (that are numbered) and after that listen for the terms that the person uses and follow his or her lead. The first five in the following list are numbered to indicate the sequence of how the layering begins.

1) Select certain brute fact and sensory experience.
2) Delete and de-select other things.
3) Foreground what you select in your mind and *background* the rest.
4) Represent that movie on the screen of your mind.
5) Edit that movie for effect.
*) Compare selected rep. against others.
*) Language it as you *classify, categorize,* and *label* it.
*) Define and *describe* a reality or concept.
*) Evaluate it as good / bad; approach / avoid; pain / pleasure and other judgments.
*) Associate it with basic emotions so that it has a particular feel, mood, or attitude.
*) Relate and *compare* it to other things with metaphors, stories, comparisons.
*) Interpret and *frame* it with higher level evaluations and understandings.
*) Set contexts and frames about it as relating it to various values and criteria.

Detecting Meaning via Meta-Questions

To begin exploring the layers of meaning, the "logical levels" in a person's Matrix of frames, the following list of meta-level distinctions gives you ten essential meta-questions by which you can discover your own or another person's layers of meaning. These ten will take you almost anywhere and are quite sufficient for anyone beginning an exploration of someone's meanings.

•	Believe	What do you *believe* about X?
•	Value / Importance	What do you *value* or find *important* about X?

- Permit, Prohibit   Do you have *permission* to do X?   Is X *prohibited*?
- Decide, Decision   What have you *decided* about X?
- Identity   *Who* are you as you X? Who would you become?
- Intention   What is your highest *intention* in X-ing?
- Metaphor (compare)   What is X like?
- Remember   What *memory* does this remind you of?
- Imagine   What do you *imagine* as you think about X?
- Expect, Anticipate   What do you *expect*?

Layered Complexity of Meaning

If you have gotten the idea that meaning is not simple, then well done! Meaning is not simple. It is everything but simple. There is complexity when you entertain the question, "What is meaning?" Yet as you been sorting out these kinds, levels, and dimensions of meaning, it does give you the ability to begin working with constructions of meaning.

Now there are several things that hclp to simplify this over-lapping mess of the different facets and encoding of meanings. The first principle for simplifying:

> *All meaning is made out of the prime components of sights, sounds, sensations, smells, tastes, etc., along with words.*

To hold any idea, thought, or awareness in your mind, you have some way to *encode* it. And when we boil meaning down to its essence, we have something in neurology, in our nervous system and brain, that we use as a symbol for something else. We use the representational system of pictures, sounds, sensations, etc.—the VAK systems (visual, auditory, kinesthetic). And to that we have words—words that label, name, and classify. And that's it. Every abstraction from these things is built up of these things frp, the various kinds of meanings. The next simplification involves the layering process:

> *All meaning involves the self-reflexivity that layers thought and feeling upon thought and feeling.*

This is the meta-stating process. You never just think a single thought, in the back of your mind you have thoughts-and-feelings *about* that single thought. Human thinking is so inevitably and inescapably reflective and infinitely so, you are forever building up incredible layers of more thoughts-and-feelings upon every awareness.

In Neuro-Semantics we often speak about this using a metaphor. It is like an onion's layers. So you may have to peel back the layers to get to the core. This is sometimes required to discover the original stimulus that sets off a whole line of thought or feeling about something.

Of course, this means that the great majority of your meanings are outside-of-consciousness. You and I are mostly unconscious of our meanings. We have habituated our naming, classifying, nominalizing, abstracting, mapping, framing, etc. to such an extent that we live inside this Matrix of our Frames of Meaning. Now that self-created Matrix *has* us. This leads to another principle:

> *All meaning is structured and involves a particular syntax.*

So the task before you is to identify that structure, find it, specify the syntax, and then check to see if it is really useful and productive, or it needs to be altered in some way. Finally:

> *All meaning is changed, altered, and transformed by meaning.*

This is the Catch-22, or paradoxical nature, of working with your meanings. When you set out to identify your meanings and enter the structured system of your meanings, you do so with a meaning-in-mind. You are seeking to do something (an intention), even if only to become aware of your meanings, and yet when you enter the system, the very act of entering changes the system. Even *you* cannot be an innocent observer in your own system! Your intentions, your understandings, your beliefs, your hopes and dreams and fears and anxieties —all of your current meanings affect how you influence your meanings.

The Psycho-Logics of Meaning

I noted earlier that Korzbyski hyphenated the word "psychology" so as to identify that every person has unique and individualized *psycho-logics*. By this he meant that *how you reason inside yourself* (your logics) *is "logical" to you and within you,* even when people on the outside may not find it logical. Whatever meaning you give to something creates a psycho-logical structure—your psycho-logics.

If you think-and-feel, and language and frame that cookies and cake are associated with feeling loved, valued, having the good life, being rewarded, and being successful— if you semantically load up cookies and cake in that way, then lo and behold, *that's what they are to you.* By association, by language, by evaluation, etc., you semantically load cookies and cake. What do they mean? Answer: All that you say they mean. Is that logical? No. But inside you it is psycho-logical. It makes sense, it is significant and meaningful to you.

Meta-Domains of Meaning

I've mentioned how that *all of the meta-levels are just different descriptions, different words, and different facets of the same thing.* This means that the so-called "logical levels" are not hierarchical. They are more like a hologram and holographical. It means that words and descriptions are redundant and over-lapping, and not different things or phenomena. You can now use this redundancy to can help you work with meaning.

In fact, there are several NLP meta-models which actually provide a redundant system of descriptions. That is, why these models seem different and approach the mind-body-system of experiences in different ways, they actually refer to the same thing. As a result they give us multiple avenues of approach. Each provides another systematic structure and description of the processes by which we construct meaning. The four meta-models of NLP are:

- The Meta-Model of Language: The NLP Communication Model.
- The Sub-Modality or Cinematic Features Model.
- The Meta-States Model of Self-Reflexive Consciousness.
- The Meta-Programs of Perceptual Lens and points of view.

1) The Meta-Model of Language

The first model of NLP, the Meta-Model is a model about the linguistics which you use to code your thoughts from the "deep structure" of your experience into the "surface sentence structure" of your words. Originating from Transformational Grammar, this model was used to sort out and model the communication patterns of Fritz Perls, Virginia Satir, and Milton Erickson.

The Meta-Model identifies the form and structure of mental mapping in terms of words and language. It unpacks the linguistic magic that governs your mental mapping and it provides you the structure of precision. From the primary representational domain of sensory-based information and language that make up the movies in your mind, you move up into the meta-linguistic domain of evaluative words.

Using this model, you can listen to words and language expressions, ask questions that invite the speaker to provide more specific answers, and in this way evoke a more thorough and precise mapping about the original experience that they are speaking about. The questions that challenge the linguistic expressions transform the evaluative language back to sensory-based words so that you can make a mental movie in your mind and understand what the speaker is referring to and hence what the person means. To study this model in more depth see the original books, *The Structure of Magic, Volumes I and II* and/or the twenty-five year update on the Meta-Model in the book, *Communication Magic*.

2) The "Sub-Modalities" or Cinematic Features Model

Classic NLP did not, and to a great extent still does not, realize that this is a meta-model. This is due to the false-to-fact term "sub" that got connected to the name. If we were to accurately label the model, it would be a Meta-Modalities model, not a Sub-Modality model.[1] This model refers to the cinematic features that encode the mental movies that you create in your mind. It refers to how you frame the cinema in your mind in terms of the qualities of your sights, sounds, and sensations. So whether you make a movie close or far, bright or dim, loud or quiet, whether you step into it or just observe it, whether you add circus music to it, or the music from Jaws, these features or distinctions enable you to be like an editor to your mental movie. And it affects your meanings.

You use these symbols to stand for some semantic evaluation. Perhaps "close, three-dimensional, and in color" stand for (and mean) "real" or "compelling." In other words, *the cinematic features* (sub-modalities) *are governed semantically.* In and of themselves, they mean nothing. Yet inside of every person, they stand for and hence encode some significance or meaning.

As you frame the cinema in your mind, you code the sights, sounds, and sensations with various features, cinematic features. These features or distinctions enable you to take *an editor's position or perspective* to your own mental movies. You can then use "close" or "far" to stand for and indicate some semantic frame (real, unreal; compelling, less compelling).

To both recognize your sub-modalities and work with these cinematic features in how you code your representations, you have to step back to observe them ("go meta"). You have to gain a broader perspective and ask questions that are *meta* to, or higher, than the representations. Is that picture close or far? Is that image bright or dim? Is that sound quiet or loud? To answer these meta-questions, you have to stop being a *subject* of the movie, step out of it, and as you transcend that experience, notice the code as it currently is. See *Insiders Guide to Sub-Modalities;* also *Sub-Modalities Going Meta.*

3) *Meta-States Mode of Self-Reflexive Consciousness*
The Meta-States Model looks at the same structures, not primarily in terms of linguistics or cinematic features, but in terms of thinking-and-feeling states. A possibility state or a necessity state, for example, will typically show up linguistically as a modal operator of possibility (can, get to, want to) and/or a modal operator of necessity (have to, must). The Meta-Model describes it linguistically, the Meta-States model describes it in terms of our experiential states.

Because you never just think, you reflectively think about your thinking, you feel about your feeling. This self-reflexivity in your consciousness creates your meta-states—your states-about-states—and enables you to do all of the layering you do on your experiences. Reflecting back onto your own states and experiences, layers levels of experiences ("logical levels") to create your unique *psycho-logics.* This means that you are not a logical creature. You are a psycho-logical being. Your meanings make sense to you—on the inside.

Nor does reflexivity ever end. Whatever you think or feel, you can step back and have another thought or feeling about that. This creates the layers of meanings as beliefs, understandings, decisions, memories, imaginations, permissions, anticipations, identities, and so on. It is what makes your mind dynamically complex and not simple. And as you continue to reflexively apply a next thought or feeling to yourself, you keep building more frames within your frame structure or matrix. This makes up the rich layeredness of your mind or your neuro-semantic system. See *Meta-States* (2008), *Secrets of Personal Mastery* (1997), and *Winning the Inner Game* (2007).

4) The Meta-Programs of Perceptual Lens

The Meta-Programs model is one of thinking patterns, thinking styles, or perceptual lens. This model refers to how you see or perceive things. Is the cup half empty or half full? Do you see it pessimistically or optimistically? Whichever style of thinking / perceiving characterizes you, then your language will differ, as will your states, as will the ways you encode your inner mental movies.

A global thinker will sort for the big picture and meta-state or frame most things from the global thinking-and-feeling state. Someone who sorts for "necessity" will regularly apply a state of compulsion to other thought-and-feeling states. Habituation of your internal processing gives rise to your meta-programs and then governs your everyday states, language, and perceptual filters. As your meta-programs show up in language, the Meta-Model offers a description. And as you access a particular experiential state and use it repeatedly, your meta-state becomes your meta-program. That's why a meta-program is a coalesced meta-state.

From your meta-states, you create the meta-programs that govern your perceptions. You generalize from the states that you most regularly and commonly access and as you do you habituate that way of thinking and feeling until it becomes your basic style of perceiving. You meta-state global thinking or detail thinking until it coalesces into your neurology and becomes your perceptual lens or meta-program. You meta-state sameness thinking or difference thinking until it becomes your meta-program style.

A *driving* perceptual style is a meta-program that you have layered with even more meta-states—states of value, belief in, identification with, etc. So if a person who thinks globally and sorts for the big picture begins to frame most things from that global state and then begins to highly value it, identify with it, believe in it, the person may create a *driving meta-program of global thinking.* Similarly the person thinks in terms of "necessity" and brings that state of mind and emotion to more and more of his or her experiences and then believes in it, values it, identifies with it, will more than likely apply that state of compulsion to every other state. This will eventuate in the *driving meta-program of necessity.*

Habituation of internal processing gives rise to meta-programs—to your structured ways of perceiving. They then govern your everyday thinking-and-feeling as your *perceptual filters.* To the extent they show up in language, you can detect them using the Meta-Model. For example, people have favored modals that describe their basic *modus operandi* (modal operators) for operating: necessity, impossibility, possibility, desire, etc. They originated as meta-level thoughts or feelings, they were first meta-states. As they coalesced, they get into your neurology, your eyes, your muscles and become your meta-programs. For more about this model, see *Figuring Out People* (2007) which is an encyclopedia of meta-programs and also *Words that Change Minds* which applies the most basic ones to the business context.

All together these four models provide four different lenses for observing your meaning-making processes.
- *Language:* Linguistics and the VAK sensory systems.
- *Cinematic Features:* The qualities and distinctions with which you code your mental movies.
- *States:* Mind-body states from which you operate.
- *Perception:* Filters for your lens for seeing and perceiving, for sorting, paying attention, and thinking.

Neuro-Semantic Learnings for a Neuro-Semanticist

What learnings and discoveries have you made from this chapter on the kinds of meanings and the NLP models that govern your understandings about meaning.

> 1) Take a meaning, something that you consider meaningful to you and begin to explore how you encode that meaning using the different kinds of meanings: representational, linguistic, evaluative. As you describe it in all of these ways, what do you become aware of?

> 2) Take a meaning that you don't like, something that bothers or upsets you and trace out its structure. As you locate the primary state experience and then move up the levels, what are the psychological levels and classifications that you discover?

End of Chapter Notes:

1. See *Sub-Modalities Going Meta* (2005) for the Neuro-Semantic approach to the cinematic features that are called sub-modalities.

2. See Dr. C.E. "Buzz" Johnson's article, "The 7, 38, 55 Myth." Anchor Point Magazine. Now posted on www.neurosemantics.com

3. This comes from *Mind-Lines: Lines for Changing Minds* (2005) and is used there to describe the linguistic model for reframing meaning and so creating linguistic influence.

4. See *Figuring Out People* (2007).

5. Where do meta-programs come from? They are mostly learned. You and I create them by meta-stating a meta-program into existence. See the chapter on the source of meta-programs in *Figuring Out People* (2007).

Figure 3:1

MEANINGS OF MEANING

Meaning takes many different forms and expression. When we ask about *meaning,* we may be asking about meaning in terms of any one of the following:

1) Origin or source, antecedent causes, beginning.
    The meaningfulness of how something started.

2) Continuity: consistency over time:
    The meaningfulness of something continuing over time.

3) Being or ontology
    The meaning of being (as existing) or in becoming (developing).

4) Identity
    The meaning of who you are, what something is.

5) Causation: antecedent causes, situational (context).
    The meaning of cause, the source of something.

6) Practicality, pragmatic, useful, or effective, real, embodiment
    The meaning of being able to make effective use of something.

7) Fantasy, imagination, openness, anticipation.
    The meaning of imagining and anticipating something new.

8) End, teleology, completion.
    The meaning of the design and end-purpose of something.

Meanings of Meaning (Continued)

9) Purpose, intention, agenda, motivation.
  The meaning of something having a purpose or design.

10) System: a network of relations, holistic, ecology.
  The meaning of the well-being and healthy of something.

11) Value, importance, axiology —Relevance to standards, criteria.
  The meaning of the value or importance of something.

12) Coherence or unity: It coheres as a meaningful pattern.
  The meaning of something having coherence.

13) Excellence, quality.
  The meaning of the quality of excellence.

Figure 3:2

LANDSCAPE OF MEANING
The Expressions of Meaning

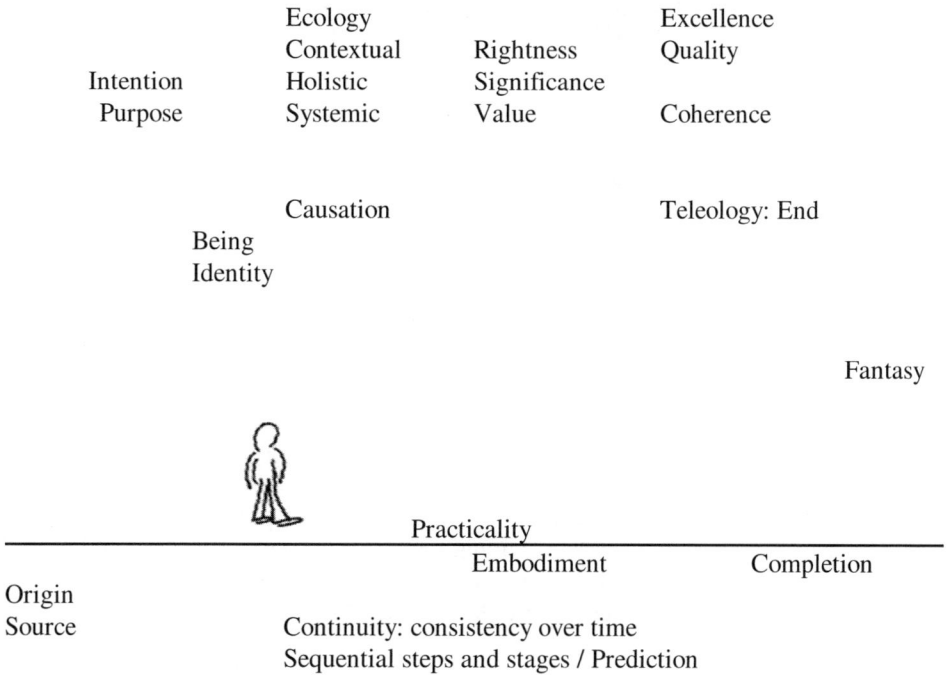

	Ecology		Excellence
	Contextual	Rightness	Quality
Intention	Holistic	Significance	
Purpose	Systemic	Value	Coherence

Causation   Teleology: End

Being
Identity

Fantasy

Practicality

Embodiment   Completion

Origin
Source   Continuity: consistency over time
          Sequential steps and stages / Prediction

Chapter 4

THE LEVELS

OF MEANING

"Structures of which we are unaware hold us prisoner."
Peter Senge

"In our brain structure, language, and perceptual systems there are natural *hierarchies* or levels of experiences. The effect of each level is to *organize and control the information on the level below it*. Changing something on an upper level would necessarily change things on the lower levels; changing something on a lower level could but would not necessarily affect the upper levels."
(Dilts, Epstein, Dilts, 1991, p. 26, *italics* added)

"Logical Levels: an internal hierarchy in which each level is progressively more psychologically *encompassing and impactful*"
(1990: 217, *italics* added)

M *eaning comes in levels.* You create meaning in levels by layering meaning upon meaning. Your meaning-making abilities begin with the sensitivity of your neurology and sense-receptors to detect that there is a world of energy manifestations "out there." That's the unspeakable level of meaning-making. In other words, *meaning begins with neurology, not cognition.*

Meaning begins with mapping to the inside that which is "out there" so that you can come to understand it and relate to it effectively. And that happens first in your body and then in your mind. So whatever is out there as the external world, whatever you say about it—is not it. Your words, as mental mapping, differ from what you are referring to. The territory is different from, and distinct from, all of your words, linguistics, and symbols. Your *map* about it is not it.

As you seek to discover what is "out there," what you are actually aware of is *the transforms* in your mind and body which your neurology and sense-receptors create. You see red and blue and green and yellow, but those are not things out there, those are effects upon your sense receptors of the energy manifestations "out there." Namely the rods and cones within your retina create your sense of color. Whatever is out there in those mysterious "energy manifestations," that science identifies as the electro-magnetic spectrum is not "color." In your processing into sights, sounds, sensations, smells and tastes you convert into the forms or maps that are meaningful to you. These are your "transforms" or mental maps—your neurological meanings.

Yet your transforms, while not the thing itself, provides you with a model or map of it. It gives you a map that enables you to relate to those sights, sounds and sensations in a way so that you can cope effectively—surviving, being safe, creating networks of relationships with others, feeling good about yourself, and unleashing your highest and best potentials. You do not have to fully or even accurately understand all that is out there, only enough so that you can use your mental models as maps to navigate the experiences that you want as you seek to enrich the quality of your life. This separates Neuro-Semantics from the other disciplines which deal with this same area: philosophy, physics, neuro-sciences, etc.

In Neuro-Semantics our focus is on *the creation of meaning*—the way we select, foreground, represent, and frame our understandings. Our focus is on modeling or mapping how a human being interprets, constructs, invents, and construes the events and people and language that we experience so that it serves us well. From NLP, we know this occurs as a systemic process of mind-body, of neurology-semantics.

Meaning is the result of what you *do* with the sensory information after you bring it into your representational awareness. I began in the last two chapters to map out, from the Neuro-Semantic perspective, how you do that at the primary level to create your associative, representative, stimulus-response, and linguistic meanings. Yet all of that is just the beginning. Meaning-making doesn't end there. Not by a long shot. In fact, from there it begins to reach for the heights of abstraction, concept, and understanding. And that's what makes us unique as a species—as infinite meaning-making creatures.

Figure 4:1

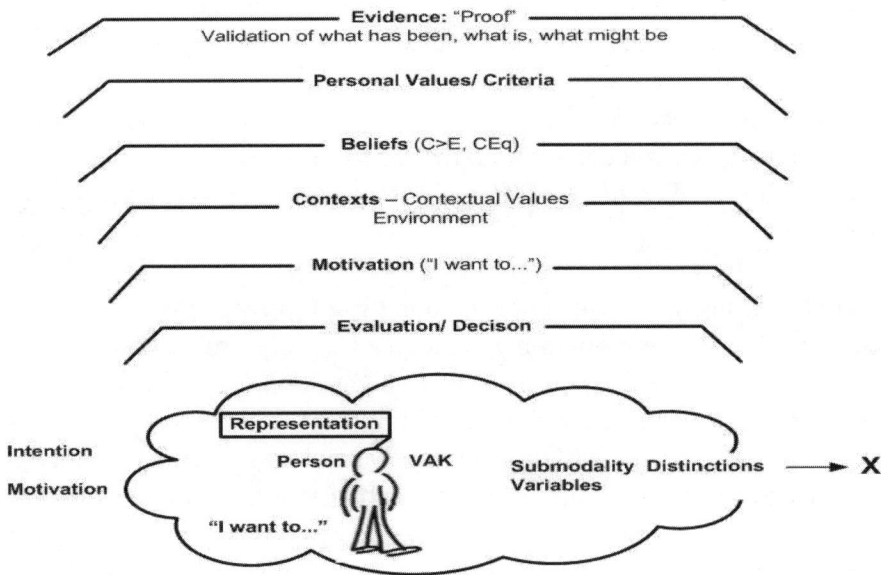

As Meaning Moves Up the Levels

Your meaning-making creativity continues as you continue to *process* the references (information) that you create. This is a function of your self-reflexive consciousness. For just as soon as you *represent* something, it becomes what you now are *referring to* (different from what that symbol stands for and refers to), you are labeling it, classifying it, categorizing it, interpreting it, and construing it to mean something. And when you create that abstract interpretation from the conclusions that you draw, the calculations you make—that then becomes the next level reference. And so it goes.

In this way you *layer* thought-and-emotion about thought-and-emotion. You create meta-states of interpretations, understandings, abstractions, decisions, memories, imaginations, intentions, etc. *layer upon layer* until you have a whole "world" or universe of meaning. This composite landscape of all your meanings we call *The Matrix* in Neuro-Semantics.

Now these *levels* that result from the *layering* are called by many names— logical levels, meta-levels, or by specific meta-terms like beliefs, understandings, memories, etc. "Logical levels" is an interesting phrase of two pseudo-nouns or nominalizations. At first it sounds like a real thing— logical levels. But what are we really talking about?

>   We are referring to *the way that you are reasoning* ("logic, logical") *and layering your reasonings upon each other* ("levels").

A logical level is not a thing. This phrase simply refers to *the process of logical layering.* Further, "logical" is a bit misleading here. That's because it is not about mathematical logic or Aristotelian logic, it is about each person's unique way of reasoning—his or her logics. So it is logical *from within* and *according to the way the person is calculating things and construing his or her reality.* From the outside it may not look or sound or seem logical at all. To describe this, Korzybski hyphenated the word psychological, to create a new term, *psycho-logical.* It makes sense to the maker of those meanings as long as he or her is living inside that construct. To one on the outside, however, it may seem more *psycho* than *logical.*[*1]

As you go up these meta-levels, *meaning grows and develops and becomes more complex.* It may also become contradictory within itself and generate internal conflict. This typically occurs because the psycho-logics you build up about one thing may contradict the psycho-logics you build up about something else. So you end up with two maps that are not congruent with each other.

>   "I want to be rich and famous; I want to live a quiet and humble life

contributing as I can."

"I want to respect and listen to what others say; I know words are just words; I will not tolerate someone calling me names. That's disrespectful and I will not stand for it. It really pushes my buttons!"

The end result is a meta-level landscape of consciousness—*your personalized Matrix of multiple frames.* This neuro-semantic landscape contains the way you have mapped concepts and conceptual meanings, culture and cultural meanings, understandings and personal paradigms, domains of knowledge and the scientific paradigms of your time and age, etc. And you do this with a thousand different things. Take anything that is very meaningful to you and you already have a matrix about it. And because of this, you can now use the Matrix Model to map out all of these meanings (see Matrix Model Questions at the end of this chapter).

Higher Level Meanings — Your Inner Frames

It is the same *reflexive process* that enables you to transform an external event into an internal representation, and then a frame of reference, that now enables you to build frames within frames. You are forever subsuming one frame within another. Reflexivity works by reflection. By reflecting on an experience, you represent it, then classify it, then frame it, and so on.

This reflexivity describes a mysterious and wondrous process. In reflecting back onto something, you step aside from it, in your mind, so that you can treat it as an object or referent. The wonder in this transcendence is that you separate the state (your thinking, feeling) from yourself. You are more than and different from your referents— your frames and even your framing.

Reflexivity within your neuro-semantic mind-body system involves a mirroring influence. Now at the primary level you do this easily as when you engage in actual reflecting as with a mirror. You reflect on your image. It is more challenging to do this mentally or conceptually because we all get so easily caught up inside of our thoughts and identify with them. Then we treat our mental mapping as real, thereby confusing map with the territory.

When you *reflect* on your thoughts *with* your thoughts, the second thoughts operate at a higher logical level than the first. In doing this, you *transcend* your first thinking. As you then think about your thoughts, your higher thoughts operate as your frame, structure, and context for the first ones. In this way *you create your own personal "logical level" system*. Each higher level functions as the class or category and the lower level as the members of that class.[2]

You start with your set of thoughts, statements, sentiments, and feelings, *about* an initial referent experience:

> Using a harsh tonality is mean.
> Only mean people speak with harshness.
> Harsh tonalities are signals that someone is going to lose control.
> Harsh tones by parents shows poor parenting.

Next, mentally *step back* from your processing and entertain your next level thoughts about them. By doing this you create meaning—a frame, an understanding, a decision, etc. You then begin to use that meaning as you refer to the experience, not realizing that you are using your constructed Matrix rather than the initial referent experience. Yet as you step back, if you transcend your current frame— knowing it is your construct—you can include it within some new conclusions that will be more resourceful:

> Those conclusions made perfect sense when I was a child of eight.
> Those conclusions reflect how scary the harsh tonality seemed to me when I was a young child.
> Those sentiments reflect poorly constructed maps.
> Such ideas do not really serve me well in terms of empowering me to cope with harsh tonalities.

You can also continue the stepping-back-reflecting process:

> Thinking through my conclusions gives me more awareness and choice.
> How I've mapped things is just that, a map. The larger question is how useful, accurate, and/or ecological the map is to my overall wealth and well-being.

Transcending and Including Infinitely

The reflexivity that allows you to shift your referent from something external to your first level representations, and then onto higher level representations, describes *the transcendence power of your consciousness.* Some of the more intelligent animals can apparently utilize this meta-function once or twice and so move up a couple of levels. Yet at some stage all animals stop. But not us humans; we never stop. For us, the reflexivity is an infinite process. For us, "the going meta" process continues without end. Whatever you think or feel about any given thought or emotion, you can then *step back* in your mind from that and think, feel, and say something about that.

What mechanism allows this? *Your use of symbols.* You can designate entirely arbitrary items to function as symbols that "stand for" something other than itself. "Mind" as intelligence, as the ability to represent, encode, decode, and function in terms of classes, sets, categories, etc., needs symbols.

Symbols free us from mere grunts, sighs, moans, growls, and other *signals.* Signals are *part of* the experience and do not "stand for" something else. Even in our communications, we present signals as part of the experience. The growl *is* the threat. The showing of the teeth *is* part of the message and action to back off. Bateson (1972) called signals, "mood signs." They are part of the state.

By contrast, *symbols free us.* In symbolic use, we can use arbitrary symbols to stand for things very different from the referent. In symbolic logic, we say that the class is not a member of the class. The class of elephants is not an elephant. The class of elephants cannot crush you or go on a rampage. The class of metal things is not a piece of metal. Conversely, the word that we use to symbolize, conceptualize, and reference a group of dogs is not a dog. "Dogs" is just a word. That term cannot bite you.

But, and this is a big neuro-semantic *but*, it is possible for you to *use* the symbol so that you can recall and re-experience a previous experience of being bitten . . . and so cue your neurology to feel the bite. This is why words and inductions are so often confused with, and believed to be, "magic." You and I can *use* language to trigger a re-experiencing of a previous experience.

As a symbolic class of life, you have a lot of latitude in your use of words as symbols. You can strictly use symbols (words, language, mathematics, poetry, etc.) as symbols that stand for other referents. And you can equally use symbols to induce or re-induce states or to even create new kinds of states.

This gives two central uses for language. You can use language to *describe* the structure of events in the world and thereby create science. You can also use language to *create* internal or neuro-semantic reality. The first one enables you to be precise, specific, and clear. It enables you to replicate your experiences and to communicate the ideas in your head. The second one enables you to be precisely vague in an indefinite way so that you can hypnotize, influence, persuade, fantasize, visualize, hope, dream, and extend the limits of human possibilities.

This is where Neuro-Semantics differs from General Semantics. Korzybski only wanted language for precision. He invented the extensionalizing devices for that purpose. He saw identification only as the misuse of the nervous system, as using the nervous system the way animals use theirs, and therefore primitive, unsane, and harmful. Yet both uses of language are legitimate especially if you know what you are doing with your words.

Neuro-Semantic Life inside of Nested Frames
So you build your layers of meanings and then you live within those meanings, that Matrix. What is that like? How does that work out?

My first answer is that most people mostly don't even know it or notice it. And why is that? *Because mental frames that set the meanings and interpretative style are mostly unconscious.* You and I live out our meanings from our frames and experience our life in terms of those frames of meaning and do so with little consciousness about it. That's why it requires some training to be able to become conscious of your frames.

My next answer is that life within your nested frames, when noticed, more often than not evokes a sense of confusion and not knowing. This occurs whenever you scratch your head and wonder:

> "Why do I do that?" "Why can't I get myself to stop doing that? I know better than that!" "What's going on, where did that come

from? I'm not like that!"

Frames govern and they govern outside-of-consciousness and so if you are conscious of them, you are conscious that there's something inside that's creating confusion, conflict, or a not-understanding. This explains one of the reasons why *frame awareness* is so often curative by itself.

The frames that you have set as you have moved through life, have the experiences that you have had, and drawn the conclusions that you have— *those frames become set as your interpretative style.* As a result this creates both a way of perceiving and a blindness to seeing in any other way. Once you live *within* your meaning frames, you no longer perceive things naively or innocently. You no longer perceive with a sensory freshness. Instead you perceive through the lens of your frames.

Your meaning frames, as you grow and they solidify, become your Matrix so that "the Matrix *has* you." It structures your thinking and feeling, it forms your expectations, it governs your responses. The meanings that you have created become your "reality strategy." And because of this, your frames operate as a self-organizing attractor. Your frames *attract* the very experiences, people, and situations that confirm its orientation, structure, beliefs, etc. Like a self-replicating DNA "code," your frames take on "a life of their own" replicating themselves in your ideas— which Richard Dawkins designated as *memes* in his 1976 book, *The Selfish Gene.*

Your meaning frames, as your code for life and reality, organizes your thinking, feeling, perceiving, acting, etc. so that the system self-organizes around those meanings. No wonder your frames attract confirming experiences and self-validate. So living in your nested frames as your landscape of meaning gives you the sense of familiarity. Your emotional sense is that things are as they are supposed to be.

Figure 4:2

————————Reference Event/ Idea/ Emotion————————

Thinking/ Representing —>

Event in
the world

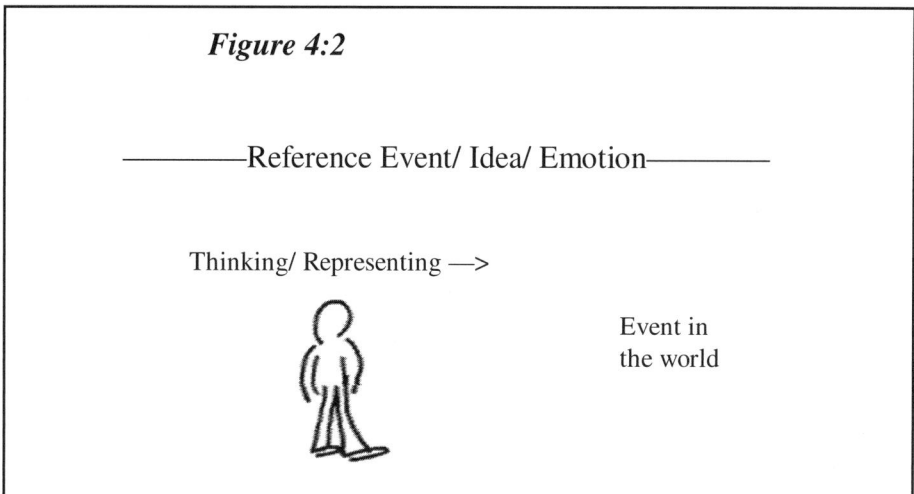

No wonder your frames are so incredibly important. Your freedom of choice, creativity, and ability to change things and experience transformation emerges from your frames. What you call a thing or person, whether "an argument" or "a search for mutual understanding," whether "a bitch" or "a person really persistent in discovering things," determines the quality and intensity of your experience.

Complexity and Hiddenness of Frames
Frames have both their public and private sides. When you first develop them, they may seem obvious to you. With habituation, however, they soon disappear from view. You forget them. As they vanish ever so slowly, you seldom notice. You simply forget that you use them as a reference, as your point of view. Eventually, you just take them for granted and assume their reality. "That's just the way it is."

Yet though you take them for granted and don't notice them, your frames will often stand out starkly to others. What seems so obvious to you seems totally ridiculous and unfathomable to others. They don't understand where you're coming from. You have to inquire, "What are you talking about?" "How does that relate to this other thing?"

This invisibility of mental frames is similar to the frames of the pictures and paintings that decorate our homes and businesses. When you are inside the picture, you don't see the frame. As picture frames disappear from perceptions and do not draw attention to itself, so our frames also disappear from our awareness.

Where do your frames go when they become invisible? Answer: They hide as a *canopy of consciousness*—the mental and conceptual world or atmosphere within which you live and move and have your being. Like the air you breathe, you also breathe in your frames as your conceptual air.

Implicit Meaning-Making

So far I've only talked about explicit meaning-making; there is also another kind, implicit meaning-making. This occurs when you construct a meaning that requires certain assumptions and presuppositions in order to make sense. But instead of making that explicit, *you just assume the meanings* that have to be in order for the things you say to make sense.

These frames, invisible to your inspection, are *frames by implication.* They imply other meaning frames. In Neuro-Semantics we often use a shorthand for these *frames by implication,* we call them FBI statements or questions. To flush out these out-of-awareness frames, ask implication questions:

- What's implied in that term, idea, or concept?
- What other implications are involved in that?
- What entailments does that metaphor carry with it?
- What do I have to presuppose in order to accept that idea?

The Experience Does Not Create the Meaning

While you think by referencing your experiences, it is not the experience that determines your beliefs, attitude, or skills. Some people experience a traumatic event like being raped, mugged, unfairly imprisoned or exiled to a concentration camp and it ruins them for life. They suffer from Post Traumatic Stress Disorder (PTSD). Others become stronger, bolder, more resolute, and enriched. Why the difference?

If the difference is not the experience, and if experience doesn't determine what you experience, then what does? Some people grow up in impoverished, toxic, and dysfunctional homes and become "victims," alcoholics, drug users, welfare cases, etc. Oprah Winfrey was similarly raped and violently mistreated in her youth. Yet today she plays a very different game. Sharing her experience, she focuses on her determination in touching the lives of millions and turning people around from victimhood.

> *It's not the experience that makes the difference, it's the frame you create about it that then sets up the game you will then play. Everything depends on the frame you set.*

Viktor Frankl noted this principle in his experience of a Nazi Concentration camp during the Second World War. Out of that experience, he set the frame that "they cannot take my ultimate freedom of choosing my own attitude." Entertaining himself with daydreams about life after the war and after the concentration camps, he went on to create an entirely new field of psychology, *Logotherapy,* the healing power of meaning. Believing that experiences do not have to control meaning, he framed the experience as something to conquer by re-interpreting them.

There are no "bad" experiences. And, for that matter, there are no "good" ones. There are just experiences. *Good* and *bad* are your judgments and evaluations about the events. These evaluation frames initiate your games that you then play. "Game" here refers to the actions and transactions that result from the frame.[3] All of your other evaluative terms that you apply to experiences, events, interactions: function/ dysfunctional; supporting/ sabotaging; traumatic/ empowering—are the *frames* that you bring to your experiences.

Now there's something truly great and wonderful about all of this:
> *Your experiences do **not** determine your future.*
> *Your interpretations are the determining factor.*

Your past experiences do **not** have the power to control your destiny or to fate you to a certain way of thinking, feeling, or acting. Above and beyond *any experience* itself is *the frame of mind* that you use to understand the experience. This also means that you can rise above your experiences. Like thousands and millions of others, you can refuse to give away your power, peace of mind, and future to a historical event—no matter how horrific or dehumanizing.

Figure 4:3

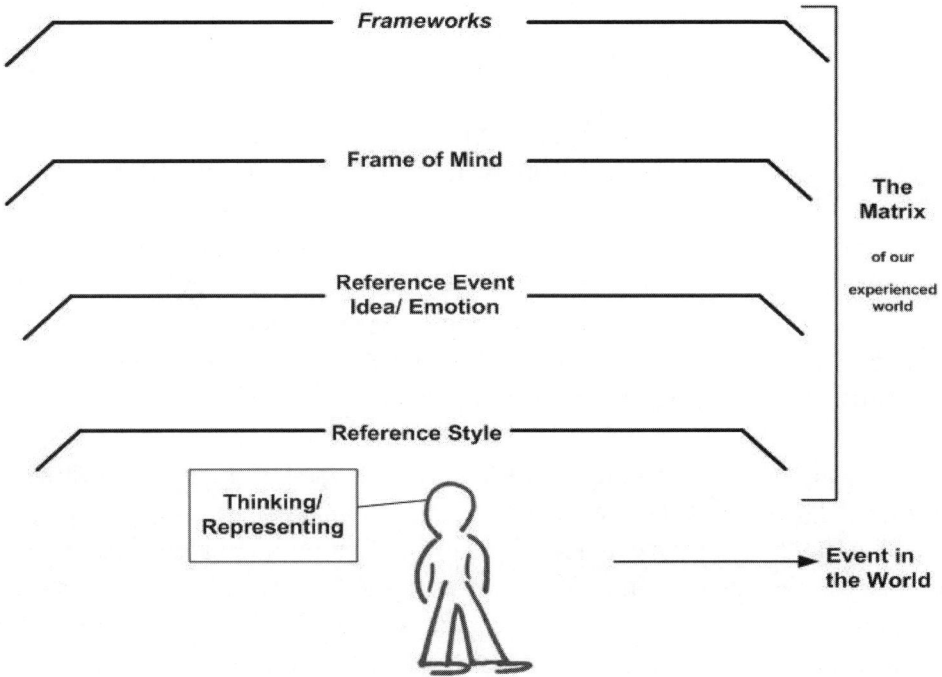

Doing that may not be easy. You may have to develop some of the *frame game skills* that you will discover in this book.[4] You may have to learn how to stubbornly refuse to buy into some default mental program for how to think about a trauma or hurtful event. You may have to learn how to utter a resounding *"No!"* to a certain frame.   After all, there are many sick and morbid frames that can undermine personal resourcefulness. And you may have to learn the mental skills of changing a frame and setting new frames.

Summary Description of Frame Development[5]
You may have to engage in some discovery of your current frames and then some analysis of what those frames have done for you.
*   What experiences have you been through?

- How have the experiences been memorable, significant, and impactful in your life?
- How have you used these experiences for good or ill?
- What games have you played, or are you playing, with those experiences?
- Do they enhance and empower you?
- What game would you be willing to play with those experiences?

What do We Call all of these Levels?

There are a lot of words we use for these levels. The most common terms are: beliefs, values, understanding, meaning, ideas, knowledge, intention, decision, etc. In Neuro-Semantics we call these terms that describe the higher levels of the mind *meta-levels* and then we explore them with questions— *meta-questions.* And each of these so-called "logical levels" are simply different terms to describe the same thing.

To understand how they all "describe the same thing," consider how they are like the facets of a diamond. Each facet on the face of a diamond is not the different thing. *Each facet is just another face or look of the same thing — the diamond.* So with meta-terms. They simply offer you another way to look at the same thing— the experience.

So if you start with the basic state of learning and you layer it with joy, that is, you meta-state the first state of learning with the second state of joy or fun or delight, then you have created *joyful learning.* Now what is this?
- Is *joyful learning* a belief? Do you believe that you can have fun learning?
- Or maybe *joyful learning* is a value. Do you value learning for the joy it creates within you?
- Is *joyful learning* a decision? Have you made a decision to have fun learning?
- Is *joyful learning* a memory? Or an imagination of your future? An expectation or an anticipation of what you have to look forward to?
- Is it an intention? Or an identity? Are you a joyful learner?
- Is it an understanding? A knowledge that you have?

So what is joyful learning? The answer is a systemic answer rather than an either-or answer. *It is all of these things at the same time– each describes the same experience from a different point of view or facet.* So is any one of these "logical levels" higher than another? Here again, you have to shift to thinking systemically rather than linearly. They are not "levels" in a hierarchical sense, they are "levels" more like the organic layering of onion layers.

Also think of these meta-states or logical levels as fluid levels that are ever in flux, ever moving. Since they are not "things," they are not rigid as the steps or stairs of a pyramid. They are more fluid than that. Each term simultaneously has within it all of the other terms so that each level can be viewed from a multiple of perspectives or facets. That's why we call the "logical levels" a *diamond of consciousness*— each offers a multi-facetic perspective.

Each of the meta-terms offers you additional ways to move around an experience. These facets give you multiple ways into the Matrix of your mind or that of another. So if you use one word or term and it does not elicit more information, use another. And when you turn them into questions, you have meta-questions by which you can explore a matrix of frames.

1. Meaning / Significance	What does this mean to you?
	What meanings are you holding in mind?
2. Belief / Believe / Confirm as real	What do you believe about this?
	What do you believe about that belief?
3. Frame / Reference	What is your frame of mind about this?
	What's your frame of reference for this?
	How are you framing this experience?
4. Permission / Allow / Permit /	Do you have permission to experience this?
Embrace / Approve	Who took permission away from you?
	Are you ready to allow this for yourself?
5. Prohibition / Taboo / Censor	Is this experience or idea prohibited in you?
	What have you tabooed?
	Who tabooed this for you?
6. Feeling (any feeling)	What do you feel about this?
	What if you could enjoy this?

	What feeling would enhance this most?
7. Thought / Notion / Idea / Word	What do you think about this?
	What thoughts come to mind regarding this?
	What's your notion about this?
8. Appreciate / Appreciation / Celebrate	What do you appreciate most about this?
	What could you appreciate about this?
	Do you appreciate this too much?
9. Value / Importance / Count	What do you value about this?
	What's important about this that you can count?
10. Decision / Choice / Will	What's your decision about this?
	What choice would you like to make about this?
	What pros and cons are you weighing?
11. Intention / Want / Desire	What's your highest intention about this?
	What do you want and really desire about this?
	What intention is driving your response?
12. Outcome / Goal / Agenda	What outcome do you have about this?
	What goal do you have beyond this goal?
13. Expectation / Anticipation	What's your expectation about this?
	What do you anticipate will happen about this?
	What do you expect about this idea?
14. Rules / Demand / Should / Must / Shall / Authorize	What *should* you do about this?
	What do you *have to* do regarding this? Why?
	What is the rule that's governing your thoughts?
	Who or what authorizes this policy for you?
15. Definition / Class / Categorize / Category / Define / Label	What definition do you use in relating to this?
	What class do you put this into?
	How do you categorize this?
	What other definition could you use for this?

Figure 4:4

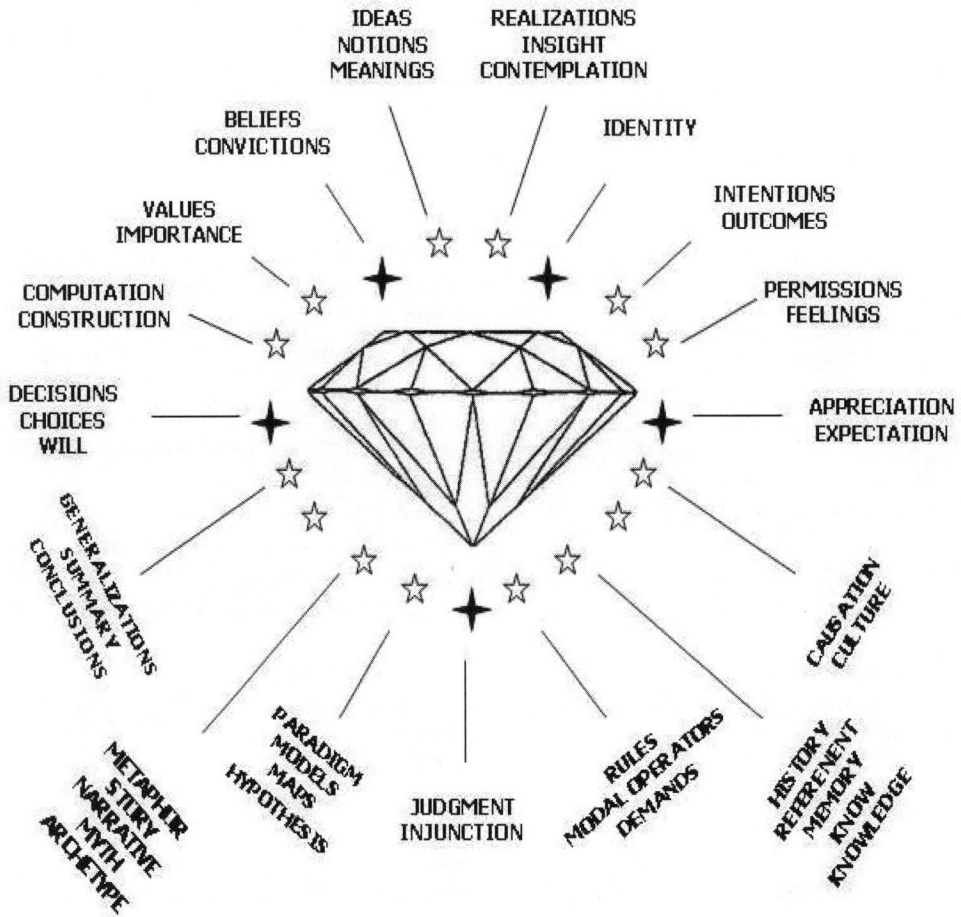

THE MATRIX MODEL

The Matrix Model combines Cognitive-Behavioral and Developmental Psychology. It is comprised of three *process* matrices and five *content* matrices. First use the *Matrix* Model as a structuring format for sorting experience out as you explore, understand, coach, manage, model, profile, and work to transform experiences. Use the specific Matrix Question to explore a Matrix, then use the model systemically for transformation.

The *process* matrices are those frames of reference, frames of meaning, and meaning constructions that we invite and then experience that make up our reality, our sense of what's real and possible.

- In everyday language, these frames are beliefs, values, understandings, intentions, anticipations, memories, imaginations, hopes, dreams, models, worries, metaphors, cultures, etc.
- Via meaning construction and intentionality, you create your mind-body-emotion *states* and experience life in those states. Yet all of this dynamic energy of meaning attribution is of your own making.

The *content* matrices are those belief frames that we build around five essential concepts that make us human beings—concepts that we never leave home without.

- Within these *content* matrices are all of our ideas, meanings, beliefs, understandings, prohibitions, rules, etc. about these given concepts or semantic realities. The five essential abstractions are *Self, Power, Others, Time,* and *the World.*

All of the sub-matrices are built around your mind-body-emotion neuro-linguistic states. What goes on at the higher levels of your meaning-making and neuro-semantic states becomes grounded in the primary states. As a model, the Matrix provides a systemic way to think about your mind-body-emotion system and how to work with it. It gives you a way to "follow the energy of information through the system" and to facilitate the enrichment of your Matrix.

The Grounding Matrix:
- **State** – the foundational matrix

The Process Matrices:
- **Meaning / Value**
- **Intention / Purpose**

The Content Matrices built around special Concepts:

- **Self**
- **Power or Resources**
- **Other or Relationship**
- **Time**
- **World**

Matrix Questions

1) Meaning Matrix:

What does it mean?
What is its significance?
What do I believe?
What do I expect?
What have I mapped about this?

2) Intention Matrix:

What do I want?
What's important?
What's my outcome?
What's the purpose?

0) State Matrix:

What state are you in?
How are you feeling?
How intense is the state?
What triggered the state?
How do you do that?
What do you call this?
What state do you have to be in to do this?
How do you get yourself into this state?

3) Self / Identity Matrix:

Who am I?   What am I like?
What's my nature?
Who can I become?

4) Power / Capacity Matrix

What should I do?   What can I do?

How should I do it?
Can I do something?

5) Others /Relationship Matrix: Who are others?
What are they like?
Are they friendly?
How can I communicate?
What do I feel about them?
How do we connect?

6) Time Matrix: Is "time" a friend or enemy?
How much do I live in the present?
How much do I live in the past or future?

7) World / Reality Matrix: What is out there?
What is real?
How does X work?
What strategy helps me deal with this?

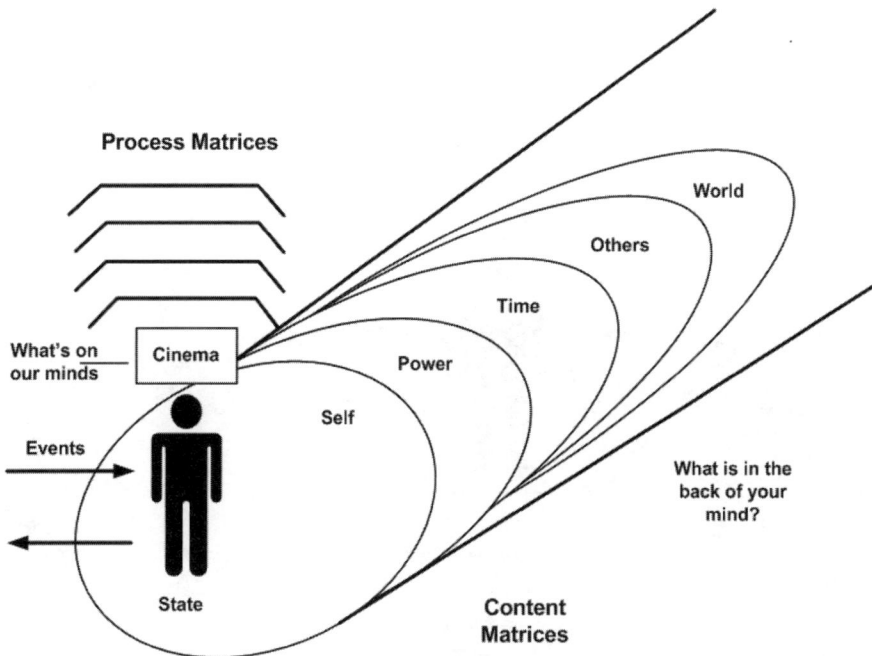

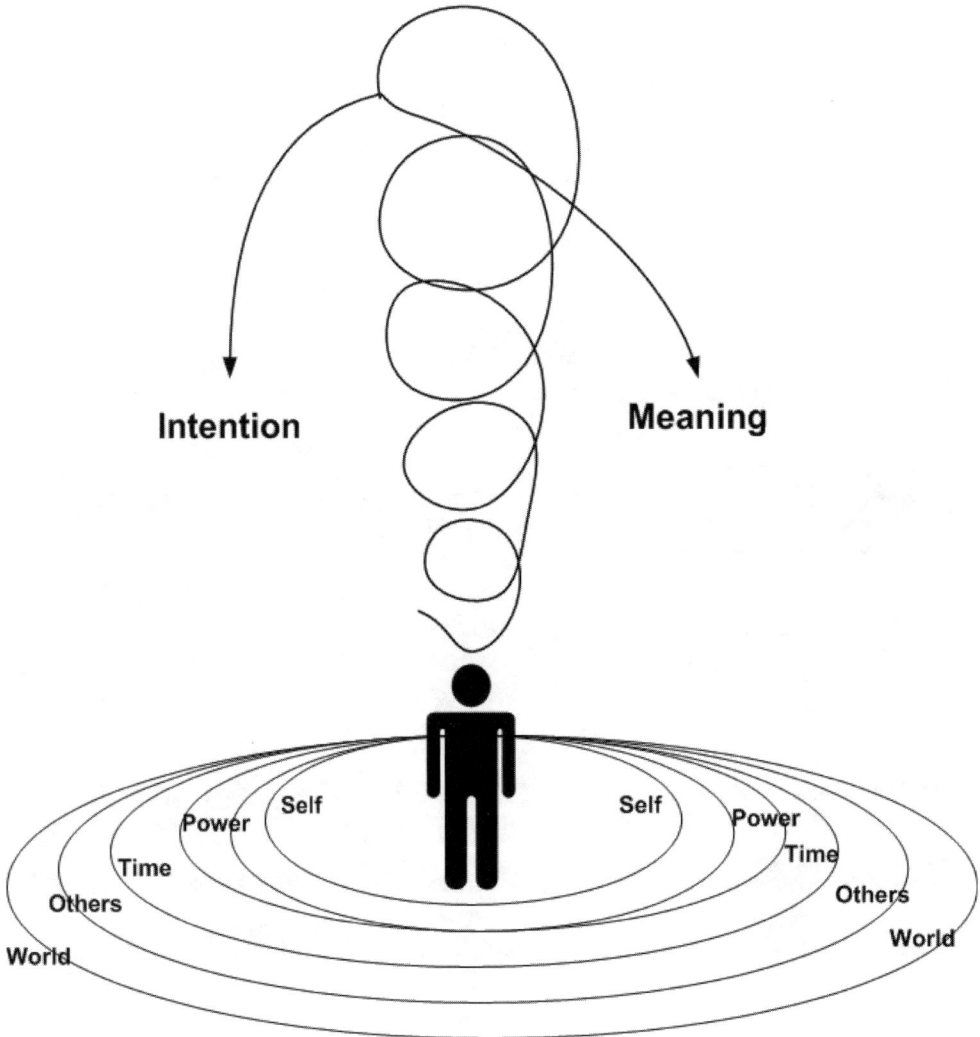

Intention

Meaning

Self   Self

Power   Power

Time   Time

Others   Others

World   World

Neuro-Semantic Learnings for a Neuro-Semanticist

Given the way your information-processing brain works, you do not just create meaning at one level, but at multiple levels. And these multiple levels of meaning frames give rise to a matrix of frames. We call these meta-levels of "logical levels" beliefs, values, understandings, and a hundred other things. And together they make up what we call "the Matrix."

> 1) How aware are you of the meta-stating that you do that sets higher level frames for your thinking and feeling? Take time this week to mentally step back from your thinking and feeling to begin to notice your second thoughts and third thoughts, etc. Doing this will be the equivalent of "taking the red pill" and discovering the Matrix you've been living in.

> 2) Sometime during the week, take one of your experiences and view it with each of the 15 meta-levels. How does that give you an expanded understanding of that experience?

End of Chapter Notes

1. This does not translate well into other languages. It is a play on the word "psycho" which in English conveys two ideas, one that of psychology and a person's psyche. The other conveying the idea of "crazy." Emphasizing that something is *psycho*-logical is a humorous play on the word.

2. I took the term "game" from the original work of Eric Bernes and Thomas Harris in Transactional Analysis (TA), as well as Timothy Gallway's work in *The Inner Game* series of books. This has led to a series of Frame Game books.

3. In his book, *Blind Elephants*, Steven Andreas has asserted that I do not believe this. Obviously Andreas has not read my original work, *Meta-States* (1994/ 2007) or he would have known that I have written about the classification and category of the higher states from the beginning.

4. See, *Winning the Inner Game* (2007), also *Games Business Experts Play; Games Fit and Slim People Play* (2001), and *Games for Mastering Fear.*

5. *Frame Games* is a user-friendly version of the Meta-States Model. In this model, the higher or meta-states are described as the *frames*—the inner context of beliefs, decisions, understandings, intentions, etc. that set up some way of acting or interacting. The *games* are the sets of actions that result from the frames. Where there is a frame, there's a game. Someone always sets the frame.

Chapter 5

EMBODIMENT

The Feel of Meaning

"Our embodiment is the key
to dealing adequately with meaning and reason."
Mark Johnson

"Meaning is shaped by the nature of our bodies,
especially our sensorimotor capacities
of our ability to experience feelings and emotions."
Mark Johnson

"Once we learn to read,
we can never again see letters as merely inky squiggles."
Daniel Gilbert

Meaning sounds like a strictly cognitive phenomenon. Yet it is not. In us humans, *meaning is an embodied experience that holistically involves our entire mind-body system.* At the very same time, meaning is both cognitive and affective. Two questions: *Is there a feel to meaning? If so, what does meaning feel like*?

In asking these questions, two answers emerge. First is that *the feel* of any particular meaning depends on the state it evokes in a person. Typically a joyful meaning elicits joy; a fearful meaning elicits fear; a meaning of sacred specialness elicits a feeling of spirituality. The second answer is that you and I feel our meanings as our emotions. That is what an "emotion" is. With this introduction, let's first explore the embodiment of meaning and then explore its manifestation as "emotion" within us.

Embodying— The Neurology of Meaning-Making

When it comes to meaning-making because you *make* meaning within, and by, your neurology (your nervous systems, brain, brain-stem, etc.), meaning is inevitably neurological. Given the kind of nervous systems that you have, you first create "meaning" in your body. Having sense receptors all over your body picking up energy signals from the world, you are actively picking up energy signals from the world. Light and sound vibrations constantly impinge upon your body. Billions of stimuli impact you, but your eyes, ears, and skin can only receive a very small amount of such stimuli. This begins the creation of your neuro-semantic reality.

Impinging stimuli is not enough. It has to *register* with you. You have to *register* it. And that's what the nervous responsiveness of your skin, sense receptors, neuro-pathways, nervous systems, etc. do. They register and record the impact of the billions of stimuli constantly impacting you.

As light and sound waves, pressure of touch, smells and tastes are then transduced from their external form, your nervous system transforms that data and converts it into another form of energy. What begins as the electromagnetic spectrum of energy manifestations ends up as bio-electric current and neuro-chemical transfer of the signal within your neuro-pathways.

This is the field and dimension of neurology. As Korzybski modeled the transfer of information through the nervous system, he referred to and developed several models. Yet his interest was not neurology, it was the larger system effect of consciousness, mind, and hence neuro-semantic reality at the everyday level.

What makes neurology important in "mind" is the fact that it orders, structures, and patterns what you experience as "information." Your nerves and nervous impulses comprise your "hardware," so to speak. The information conveyed through and by your neurology occurs at a specific rate, approximately 120 metres per second. Information also occurs in specific parts of the body and brain. Nerve impulses enter the body as the sense receptors and then travel to the lower centers of the brain, the brain-stem, thalamus, and then on to the higher centers, the cerebral cortex where it is processed by higher associative parts of the brain.

You experience the energy manifestations "out there" in terms your "senses," that is, vibrations, movements, and bodily energies. The stimulations "out there" are mechanical impacts that you abstract inside your body and experience as tactile sensations such as pressure, rhythm, movement, etc. You experience mechanical vibrations of the air as "sound." If the vibrations register within a range from 30 to 30,000 or even 50,000 vibrations a second, it is sound. Above or below that range and you hear nothing.

You experience the vibratory manifestations of electromagnetic waves as "light." Your nervous systems, however, can only register a very limited range, namely, the waves called radiant heat and light waves. You can register another form, the ultra-violet rays, but only on a chemical level. You have no sense-organ that can directly register electric waves, ultra-violet rays, X-rays, and many other rays. You also experience the chemical "senses" of taste and smell. Yet you register only a very small number of excitations.

Korzybski (1933/ 1994) wrote,
> "... structurally we are immersed in a world full of energy manifestations, out of which we abstract directly only a very small portion, these abstractions being already colored by the specific functioning and structure of the nervous system" (p. 238)

From Vibration Energy to Nervous System Impulse Energies
The energy manifestations "out there" beyond your nervous system enter within your body via your end-receptors and becomes a "nervous impulse" that travels through brush-like connections (synapses) and along a nerve-fibre as it transmits the energy now in the form of the impulse. As it moves through the reflex circuit, there are many different kinds of nerve cells that

process it. It moves through the estimated twelve thousand millions of nerve cells (neurons) in the brain, more than half of which are in the cerebral cortex. As it does this, it generates different kinds of responses. Nerve cells can excite, inhibit, diffuse, etc. Nervous functions in your body involve such responses as irritability, conductivity, integration, etc.

Because it *responds,* living tissue is alive. The foundation of biology (the study of bio, *life*) lies in the dynamic nature of protoplasm that we call irritability. Touch organic material and it reacts. Living cells have a relationship to the environment and to external energies because of their limiting surface. This creates a difference between what's "inside" the skin and what's "outside." Structurally, it establishes boundaries, borders, membranes, transfer of energy, the interplay between environment and organism, etc.

With living tissue, there's an excitation-transmission gradient. This is the basis and origin of your nervous system. Nerves become "structuralized and permanent physiological gradients and so exert a physiological dominance over other tissues" (Korzybski, p. 104).

Living tissue also reflect electrical structures so that it transfers bio-electrical currents. This is no surprise given that neurology represents electrical structures. Electrical charges that repel and attract establish order, structure, rhythm, etc. in the body so that your "mind" ultimately has a physico-electro-chemical structure.

Not only is there *order* in how your nervous system operates, as it operates, it does so in an ordered way. It operates cyclically and holistically. The nerve impulses not only move linearly in a certain direction, the impulses also travel in cycles and loop around a circuit. The interconnectedness of the brain makes it a system, a brain-body system that works as a whole (holistically). This means that the nerve impulses that carry the signals, which you and I eventually experience as "information," is *processed* repeatedly, at different stages along the way. Suppose we asked the linear, either-or question, "What part of the brain is involved in seeing? It is due to "sense" or to "mind?" This misleads and misunderstands the holistic nature of the brain. Structurally, "seeing" results from a cyclic interdependent process of both the lower and higher parts of the brain.

Your nervous tissues becomes organized for this transform of information in all of these (and many more) ways, giving form, order, structure, etc. to the data because it is comprised of protoplasm. And protoplasm, by its very nature, is responsive to the world. Korzybski said that "all living protoplasm 'abstracts'" (p. 166). That is, it registers, translates, and conveys information. That's why he made *abstracting* fundamental for "intelligence" and "mind."

> "If we speak in neurological terms, we may say that the present nervous structure is such that the entering nerve currents have a natural direction, established by survival; namely, they traverse the brain-stem and the thalamus first, the sub-cortical layers next, then the cerebral cortex, and return, transformed, by various paths." (Korzybski, 1994, p. 169)

This establishes the basis for how *structure* plays a critical role in mind and meaning. The structure of your nervous system establishes that you experience your "senses" first and then "mind." In Neuro-Semantics (as in General Semantics) we use this to establish the difference between two kinds of *mind-states:* those that we call "emotions" from those that we call "rationality" or "thinking." Both are mind-states generated by the nervous system and brain and are embodied within the same nervous systems. One represents the lower brain centers (thalamus, hypocampus, etc.), the other represents the higher brain centers, the more elaborate processing that occurs in the cortex.

> "Since the cortex has a profound influence upon the other parts of the brain, the insufficient use of the cortex must reflect detrimentally upon the functioning of the other parts of the brain. The enormous complexity of the structure of the human brain and the corresponding complexity of its functioning accounts not only for all human achievements, but also for all human difficulties." (Korzybski, 1994, p. 178)

"Mind" Neuro-Semantically

We take it that "mind" and "meaning" emerge from within your unique neuro-linguistic system. That is, that these experiences are emergent properties that arise in your mind-body system. "Mind" *is* not the brain. It arises from the way your brain *processes* information given the kind of body and nervous system you have, given the nature of physics in the kind of world you live within. "Mind" is not the ghost in the machine. It is not a non-physical entity like a spirit or demon that enters the system from without. It *emerges* from within —from the functioning of the neuro-semantic system.

Cognitive linguists (Lakoff and Johnson) speak about mind-body and the body-mind and hence *embodiment*.[1] Embodiment means that your sense of the world, yourself, each other, and the way you language things (since all languaging is metaphorical) arises to a great degree from the kind of embodiment you have given the kind of body you live in.

Embodying — The Creation of "Emotions"
The feel of meaning inevitably shows up as emotions in your body. Emotions are secondary to meaning because they are derived from meaning. Meaning is primary. In fact, until you know what something means, you won't know what to feel. If you don't know what it is, what it lead to, what it causes, how you evaluate it, the value you endow it with, and so on—you won't know what to feel.

Now in speaking about emotions, I'm not speaking about sensations or feelings. Those are kinesthetic sensations which you experience in your body. And while they certainly are a facet of an emotion, they are not emotions. Breathing hard, eyes dilating, hands sweating, heart pounding, adrenal glands secreting— these are sensations, feelings, and kinesthetics. From these same feelings, numerous emotions emerge—anger, fear, excitement, or lust.

The determining factor if these sensations contribute to any one of those four emotions *depends on your thoughts* by which you create your emotions. If you evaluate your situation as one of threat, danger, or challenge—the emotion could be fear or anger and that depends upon your learning history as well as your current evaluation as to whether you can handle it or not—*anger* if you can, *fear* if you cannot. Anger moves you toward the source of the threat; fear moves you away from it. If your thoughts create within you a mental context of desire, if the desire is sexual, then you experience *lust*. If it is a general desire for something that you highly value, then *excitement.*

And as you will later discover, the additional layers of meanings that you give to any one of these emotional states will layer additional texture and quality to the emotion that you experience. So how do you *feel* your meanings?

> *The feel of meaning inevitably shows up as emotions in your body.*

> *You feel them in your body as you somatize your meanings and transform them into what we call emotions.*

So whatever emotion you experience, whatever emotional state you access and experience—*your emotion is a function of your meanings.* That explains why you can learn to detect, monitor, and manage your emotions by detecting, monitoring, and managing your meanings. Your emotional responses is a symptom of your meanings. You can now use your emotions as symptomatic indicators or expressions that tell you what something must mean to you. And if you have a problem with an emotion— the problem is not really with the emotion, it is with the meaning that's generating that emotion and probably with the meaning you give to that experience.

It should therefore be no surprise or marvel that you then somatize or embody your meanings so that they become your emotions and expressed through your actions and behaviors.

In transforming a meaning into an emotion, the term "emotion" tells the story. The word itself refers to "moving" (motion) "out" (ex) from where you are to somewhere else. Thus an e(x)motion is defined in any classic psychology book as "an action tendency, an activation of the motor cortex." *Emotions create motion within you, motion to move, to do something, to make some action.* Emotions provide you the energy to act on your meanings.

In Neuro-Semantics we define an "emotion" as *the difference between your mental model and your experience in the world.* This definition focuses on the dynamic inter-change between two phenomenon— your map about things and your experience of those things. And the most relevant metaphor that provides a word picture of this is a balancing scales.[2]

On one side of the scales is your mental world and inner game of the meanings that you give to things, the meanings of what something is, how it works, what you expect, etc. Over against that is your actual experience in the world, how you are actually acting and experiencing the territory that your map describes. If map and experience of the territory balance out so that they are about the same—so that what you thought, expected, understood, etc. is happening in how you are coping, then there's not a lot of emotion or energy.

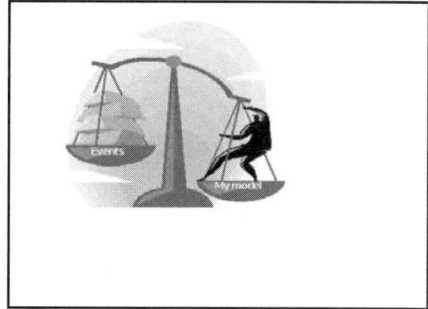

But if your experience in the world is *not* living up to your mental mapping of that world, then the scales tip downward on the territory side and generate what we call the "negative" emotions. They are negative in that they are inhibitory and provide various warnings that something is wrong. And what's wrong? Somehow the world is wrong in terms of your map. The world is not living up to your map. And the more it is wrong, the more this generates increasing levels of emotion– anger, fear, sadness, stress, distress, shame, guilt, etc.

If these emotions continue to warn that there's something not-right about how you are coping with the world, and for all of your shifts and changes in your adaptation to reality out there, then an even more frightful thing arises— maybe your map is wrong! After all, the world of events and people keep violating your map.

If, however, your experience in the world seems to be working, what you mapped out and expect and understand is coming true so that the way you are coping with things is working, then the scale tips upward and you experience what we call the "positive" emotions—joy, happiness, love, contentment, passion, compassion, tenderness, appreciation, etc. And this provides energy to keep doing what you are doing that seems to be working.

The emotions that we call the positive emotions *validate* your map and your coping (acting) and so encourages you to continue. The negative emotions *invalidate* your map and/or your coping and move you to stop, look, and listen" and make changes. Something is not right somewhere and something needs to change.

> *Your emotion is a function of your meanings.*

Emotions as the Embodiment of Meaning

As you create "meaning," it is not only intellectual or cognitive, it is neurological as well. It involves your physiology. It is behavioral, emotional, and somatic. And the first and inevitable embodiment of your meanings occurs in your emotions.

One way that we express this in Neuro-Semantics is to say that *we metabolize our thoughts and meanings.* That is, just as you breathe and take in food and then metabolize the oxygen and nourishment so that you transform it into your body— into organs, bones, muscles, skin, eyes, hair, etc., so you also metabolize thoughts. You take in words, ideas, representations, interpretations, concepts, etc. and you *process* what nourishes your mind and spirit and so metabolize it into your body as your emotions, your patterned behaviors (habits), linguistic pattens, etc.

Metabolizing meanings is the embodying process that literally incorporates what you think and believe into your body. "Corp" is another word for body and the term *in-corporation* speaks about how you make a conceptual understanding part of yourself. It becomes "installed" as a "program" that governs how you operate.

We see this metabolizing process in what we call "habits." By habituating a set of thoughts, beliefs, or actions, by the repetition you make your understanding part of your automatic response pattern. Now it "drops into your unconscious mind" and operates apart from your conscious awareness. Now you can continue to use your neuro-pathways and generate behaviors in a way that indicates the meanings that inform those behaviors are now fully embodied. This is what makes your life truly *neuro*-semantic.

The importance of this is that by embodying your meanings, then your meanings form and govern your physiology and embodied experiences. This enables the meanings to become *real* and *authentic* in actuality and not merely in thought and conception.

State— An Embodiment and Grounding of Meaning

Given that you embody meaning and feel them in your emotions—*an emotional state embodies and grounds your meaning.* If I were to express the opposite of this, I'd say: If your meanings are not putting you into a mind-body-emotion state, you have not yet embodied those meanings or integrated those meanings.

State is what makes your meanings real in yourself, in your body, and therefore in your actions and what you actually do in the world. State is the actualization of the meanings that you create at all levels of your mind. I didn't know that when I first began elaborating the structure of the Meta-States Model. At first I didn't know how to "anchor" or integrate a meta-state so that it would be registered at the kinesthetic level. Yet it wasn't long before I discovered that meta-states are constantly being embodied—integrated and actualized in the primary state where they can be anchored by a touch.

The event that changed my mind was a conversation with a young man whose meaning-making involved constructing an identity of "being a failure." Now "failure," as an abstract concept coded as a nominalization, is itself a linguistic muddle. That's why, using the Meta-Model of Language we first de-nominalize it by indexing its references:

> What did you fail out? How did you fail? To what extent? What criteria are you using to compare the event against and make the evaluation that you have failed to achieve some objective? Does anything stop you from learning from what didn't work and resiliently giving it another go?

As a short and quick way to drive home the point that *failure* does not exist "out there," but is a judgment of the mind, I asked, "Where do you feel this failure?" As I asked that, I expected that he would have to answer as everyone else that I had asked the question did, "Well, I don't feel it in my body, it is my evaluation of things." Instead, his answer surprised me. "Right here!" he said as he pointed to the pit of his stomach

> An emotional state embodies and grounds your meaning.

and using the fist of his right hand to push into his stomach as if it was hitting himself.

I was shocked. I didn't expect that at all. When I explored further, it turned out that as a child, when his dad would become upset or angry with him, he would take it out by literally punching him in the stomach and saying:

> "You're such a failure, I can't believe you are a child of mine, what's wrong with you? You're always going to be a failure acting like that!"

No wonder the meaning-making of the young man was now anchored to, and incorporated in, a punch in the stomach! And no wonder he embodied the thoughts-and-feelings of his evaluative judgment about "being a failure" to the neurology and physiology of feeling punched and doubling over. He had thoroughly metabolized his meanings, incorporated them, and habituated them until they were well anchored.

Dis-Embodying Toxic Meaning

So what can you do when a toxic meaning like, "I'm a failure," gets embodied in neurology? Can we get that meaning of the body out? Can we expel it so that we no longer feel things in that way?

The good news is *Yes we can!* After all, even your neurological state is a dynamic one—ever changing. It is not the case that once you create it, you are stuck with it. After all, everyday you are sending messages and commands to your body via your neuro-pathways. So to change an embodied felt-meaning that's been somatized, you first have to identify and interrupt the current messages and messaging that you are engaged in. Then you can replace those signals with more appropriate and useful ones. What patterns can you use to do this? (You can find these in the later chapters).

- The Drop-Down Through Pattern (chapter 13)
- The Crucible Pattern (see *Unleashed!* 2007)
- The Matrix Coaching Pattern (chapter 14)

Belief Embodiment

One of the most important things I learned during my time with NLP co-founder Richard Bandler was the distinction he made about beliefs. While thoughts obviously send messages to your body, they are just that, *messages*. Beliefs, however, are different. *Beliefs send commands to the nervous system*.[3] That means that a belief's power as a self-fulfilling process operates by setting a higher level frame that governs all subordinate experience.

Now systemically, when a state moves to a higher level, a gestalting process occurs so that the meta-stating becomes something "more than the sum of the parts" (the literal meaning of the term *gestalt*). When you meta-state a thought and layer it with other thoughts-and-emotions, it becomes a gestalt, what we call a *belief*. A *belief* is a confirmation thought about a thought; it arises when you bring *confirmation (validation)* to a thought frame it as "real, true, the way things are," etc. And as a belief, this higher level meta-state becomes a command to the nervous system instructing your body and neurology how to respond and what to do.

In terms of meaning-making and the embodiment of meaning, this is another central way that you embody and integrate higher level meanings (concepts, abstractions, understandings, decisions, identities, etc.). You *believe*. When you believe in a meaning you begin a process whereby you embody that meaning thereby making it real in your body. You set an executive order in your body that operates as a self-organizing attractor so that it self-organizes you to the content of the belief.

Quality of Meaning — The Quality of Life

Why is all of this about embodiment important? *Because the quality of your meanings is the quality of your life.* You can have no higher quality of life than the quality of your meanings. So creating rich and robust meanings is the process for how you can improve the quality of your life. I'll add one more thing, from the Psychology of Self-Actualization. Namely this—you and I have within us *a self-actualization drive.* Your mind-body system is designed to *actualize* the messages it receives. That is the process. Now *what* it actualizes is whatever you commission to make real in your mind-body.

> A *belief* is a confirmation thought about a thought; it arises when you bring *confirmation (validation)* to a thought frame it as "real, true, the way things are," etc.

From Neurology to Semantics

So what is meaning? And where is it? These are not easy questions to answer. Answering these questions involve much complexity. And there's a simple reason for this complexity: meaning is made by people who are themselves complex in how they make meaning. Because you invent meaning in many ways and at different levels, you do so using your own self-reflexivity and psycho-logics.

In review, you have to make meaning because, apart from bringing your "mind" to the events and experiences of life— there is no meaning. Meaning arises as your interpretation, understanding, and construction. It is your feeling and sense of significance. And because without your intervening neuro-linguistic state, there is no meaning. Meaning arises from the working of your neuro-linguistic states.

Because you are essentially and inescapably a meaning-maker, to make sense of life and experiences, you find and create order, structure, and patterns. The patterning and structuring that you create about things is what we call "meaning." And these patterns you "hold" in mind. You pattern and order meaning in your mind-and-body. All of this raises lots of questions about the semantics by which we live your life:

*   What makes meanings meaningful?
*   What makes meanings significant, worthy of investment, valuable, and important?
*   What matters most to you? Health (fitness, energy, vitality), responsiveness, beauty, integrity, resilience, creativity, learning, responsibility, respect, honesty, being forthright, etc.

Here's another complexity. While we typically think of meaning as "thoughts," and therefore mental and conscious, that's only part of the story. Meaning begins much lower. In making sense of things

> *The quality of your meanings is the quality of your life.*

you generate your meanings from the body upward. As you do this, you begin with meaning that is non-conscious and pre-conceptual—at the bodily level of your neurology. The first meanings you make are non-propositional and non-linguistic. In this your body "abstracts" (make summaries and draw conclusions) about things and from that level of neurological abstracting, all of the next levels of abstracting arise. Mark Johnson (2007) writes:

> "Mind is an achievement, not a pre-given faculty. Meaning requires a functioning brain, in a living body that engages in its environments— environments that are social and cultural, as well as physical and biological." (p. 152)

First stages: Embodied meaning in Neurology:
  1) Neurological embodied knowing non-conscious knowing.
  2) Felt meanings: knowing through the senses, felt patterns like "balance," "up," and "out."
  3) Experiential knowing: actions, habituation, domains of experiences, associative meanings.
  4) Procedural knowing: know-how causation, non-propositional process meaning, pragmatic.

Second stages: Embodied Meaning in Semantic Awareness
  5) Sensory representational knowing: associative meanings.
  6) Linguistic meanings: using various meta-representational systems for knowing: defining, classifying, identifying, inferring, conceptualizing.
  7) Conceptual meaning: metaphorical, theoretical, causation, abstract propositions.
  8) Significance knowing: values, importance.
  9) Intentional knowing: purpose, direction, teleological.
  10) Environment and cultural knowing: cultural beliefs.

If we stretch meaning-making out on a continuum, it would cover the area from body to mind, from performance to conceptualization, from doing to knowing. And if we divide the continuum in half at the mid-point, that would give us the Meaning — Performance Axes.

Figure 5:1

Meaning	Performance
Mind-Semantics	Body-Neurology
Environment/ Culture Significance	Neurological felt meanings
Conceptual - Linguistic - Representational Intentional	Experiential - procedural

---

When you order, pattern, and structure things in this way, you create a coherent and comprehensive experience, a mapping that gives order to life. As you *select* certain features to attend to you *de-select* many other things. The end result enables you to create a network of meanings—the Matrix Model. You create a meaningful coherent unity in your mind by organizing mental representations with an order. This creative act brings something new into existence— your personalized map of reality.

All of this generates the semantic phenomena that you then live with, and operate from. In these ways you create your mappings that enable you to explain things to yourself and invent ways to deal with those realities. In describing how you process or "bring information in" from the world via your neurology and then your mind, Alfred Korzybski called this abstracting.

Neurological Levels of Meaning-Making

1) Neurological embodying of meaning

To know something neurologically is to know it in your body, as you know "balance" via your vestibular system. This contributes to your orientational awareness of where you are in space. At this level you know in perception via perceptual acts. Meaning is first shaped by the nature of your body, especially your sensorimotor capacities and your ability to experience feelings and emotions.

2) Felt meaning

Mark Johnson refers to many of the domains of experiences that you know at a pre-conceptual and pre-cognitive level:

in/out	balance	time/ temporality	monetary transactions
traveling	journal	building things	forces and energies
connection	seeing	center/ periphery	grasping
up/down	paths	links	scales

John Grinder calls this level "first access." Meaning grows from your visceral connections to life and your bodily conditions of life. Movement itself is part of the foundational basis for meaning. Meaning is not just what is consciously entertained in acts of feeling and thought, meaning reaches down into your corporeal encounter in your environment.

3) Experiential meaning

To know experientially is to know through the experiences you have as you engage and interact with the world.

4) Procedural meaning

This is your know-how knowledge, your pragmatic procedural knowledge, "What I can do with X?" Know-how refers to the knowledge of how things work and how to do things with that knowledge.

5) Representational knowing

This is the sensory knowledge that you experience as you perceive visually, auditorially, kinesthetically, and by all of your other senses.

This is your code knowledge that makes up the languages of the mind." Representational knowledge is covered in NLP by the representational systems, the Strategy model, and the Meta-Modalities (or sub-modalities) model.

6) Linguistic knowing

In early NLP Bandler and Grinder called this the Meta-Representational system.[4] It refers to your classification knowledge what you know by definition that something is, its identification. It refers to how you understand things by language. This level is covered in NLP by the Meta-Model of language, the Milton Model of hypnotic language patterns, and by the Mind-Lines Model.

7) Conceptual knowing

This is the theoretical knowledge that involves your inferences and higher cognitive functions. This knowledge is about what causes things to work (causation). It enables you to build an explanatory system for things. What is happening, what happened, will happen? With an explanatory system you are able to make sense of things. How well does your concepts correspond to the territory that you are mapping. This includes abstract knowledge that you create through cognitive extension and projection. This level is covered primarily by the Meta-States Model along with the Meta-Programs Model, the Self-Actualization Quadrants, and the Matrix Model.

8) Significance meaning

This refers to your knowledge about why X is important and the significance you find in it or that you attribute to it. This level of meaning formulates the value and richness of life. This level is covered by Meta-States Model along with the semantic Meta-Programs Model, the Mind-Lines Model, the Self-Actualization Quadrants, and the Matrix Model.

9) Intentional knowing

Your knowledge about why you do X, or purpose, and direction, your intention that leads to commitments and engagements.

Intension creates your focus. This is covered by Meta-States Model, the Self-Actualization Quadrants, the Intention Matrix in the Matrix Model.

10) Environmental and Cultural knowing

The meanings that you "absorb" from and within your environments and especially in your cultural environments. This level is covered by the Meta-States Model, the Self-Actualization Quadrants, and the Meta-Modeling of Neuro-Semantic Modeling Model.

Meaning — Up From the Body

We create meaning from the body upward. Meaning-making begins from the body due to its neurological qualities, mechanisms, and functions. You have no other option but to make meaning using your body. In making this point in *Science and Sanity* (1933/ 1994), Alfred Korzybski came up with the two terms—*neuro*-linguistics and *neuro*-semantics. What he wrote has now become the foundational knowledge in the neuro-sciences, namely that what is "out there" in the world is the electromagnetic spectrum of energies and when our neurology experiences it, we experience it in terms of the constructs that we create in our bodies as light, sound, and sensation. We transform the energy out there and so it shows up in neurology as the things we see, hear, feel, and so on.

Take color as an example. What does *color* mean? If you make meaning about color *from the body upward*, then you first look at your neurological meaning-making and your semantic and linguistic meaning-making. So you begin with the rods and cones in the structure of your eyes. This structure translates, interprets, distorts, abstracts, and changes the energies "out there," and transduces that information so that you experience it as color. You see red, green, blue, yellow, and so on. Color exists for you because of the way your eyes work. It arises in your experience due to how your eyes are structured.

Color is therefore meaningful to you because it is a way that you have in your neurology to distinguish things "out there." This allows you to categorize things (red things, blue things, black things, etc.). That's how it starts. From there you give different colors other kinds of meanings.

"Warm" colors, "cool" colors, "pretty" colors, "ugly" colors, etc. You relate colors to states, emotions, and all kinds of things. What does any given color mean? It depends on what you or someone else connects it to. The *body* part of the meaning gives the color experience and the *mind* part of the meaning depends on the language system, personal associations, and cultural beliefs.

This shows how "color" has meaning from the body up to your highest abstractions of concepts, beliefs, and belief systems. Once you have the experience, you develop beliefs about colors and so you given more value and importance to some colors than to others.

So while meaning starts to be constructed in the body via your neurology, it does not end there. Once the fundamental levels of meaning rise to consciousness, "mind" takes it from there and creates prolific meanings. Given the kind of bodies that we have and the nature of our bodies, the fundamental levels give you the basis for your meaning-making.

This is what George Lakoff and Mark Johnson in Cognitive Linguistics have worked on for several decades. In *Metaphors We Live By* and *Philosophy in the Flesh* they documented how body and physiology enter into the meaning-making process. They point out that the fact that your body stands erect gives the metaphors of "front" and "back" thereby leading to our basic orientation in the world. As we "face" things literally to move, so we "face" things in our thoughts, emotions, and experiences.

We look at other things in terms of "before" and "after" —straight ahead and behind, up and down, right and left. The elemental orientation meanings arise from your body and then is cultivated by your consciousness to create your first and basic metaphors, the metaphors that you *live*. Given that your body is a container, you have a sense of what is "inside" and "outside." That you go inside of buildings and come out of them, all of these physical facets of experiences intimately influences your language and your semantics. You *live* "going forward," "facing" life and people. You live trying to move *up* to the next level, experiencing "move" and "up" and "less" as down. You live in the idea of boundaries, going "in" and "out" of things and ideas.

So the life that you live *in* your body and *from* your body makes your body the instrument that you use to "make sense" of life as you know it. First your body senses the world— it smells, tastes, feels, etc. You sense the world via your sense-receptors: eyes, ears, skins, tongue, nose, inner ear, stomach. These neurological and physiological experiences become *metaphors* for how your senses an make sense of other things.

So What?

One significance of this is that all of your meaning-making is connected. That's why I made the list of neurological and semantic meaning-making factors or mechanisms. These factors lie along a continuum. Why is that important? Because if they are connected, then the Mind-to-Muscle pattern enables you to move *down* to more specific and body-facets of meaning to *embody* the meaning in your neurology, in your muscles, in your neuro-pathways, in your organs.

This also provides some of the theoretical background that legitimizes the translation of meaning from one level to another level. It means that thinking as movie-making and then self-reflexive thinking as meta-stating is our primary way for moving up the levels. It suggests that we can create other mind-to-muscle processes which will be of much more value to people, companies, businesses, education, etc.

The bottom line is that *mind emerges.* It emerges from brain, brain structures, and the nervous systems govern your body, physiology, and neurology. We begin here. We begin with the basic responsiveness of the nervous system to the energies in the world.

Neuro-Semantic Learnings for a Neuro-Semanticist

Meaning isn't just a cognitive phenomenon. It originates as a neurological phenomenon and even as the higher levels of your cortex articulates meaning cognitively, it then sends it back down into the body as muscle memory and action readiness. As you now reflect on your learnings from this chapter, here are some questions:

> 1) Begin with a diagnosis to detect where you are today in terms of embodying your meanings. What meanings have you embodied? How well are those meanings serving you?

2) Now that you know about how you embody meaning, what meanings would you like to commission your body to "know" and experience? Make a list of some great meanings that you have made intellectually that you are ready to integrate into your body.

3) What meanings have been embodied that you need to release and deframe and get out of your body? What meanings lower the quality of your life and diminish the quality of your life?

End of Chapter Notes

1. See the works of Cognitive Linguistics George Lakoff and Mark Johnson for extensive and well documented studies on embodiment.

2. For more about emotions in Neuro-Semantics, see *The Sourcebook of Magic* (1977) chapter 6. Also see *Unleashed* (2007) chapter 11.

3. This statement comes from the book, *Using Your Brain — For A Change* (1985) by Richard Bandler.

4. See *The Structure of Magic, Volume I* (1975).

THE QUESTIONS OF MEANING

Meaning as Why

Why are we here?
Why are we doing this?

Meaning as Where

What is our purpose or cause?
What difference will this make?
What value or significance will it have?
What is our intention?

Meaning as What

What is this? What else could it be?
What is our identity? What is our history (continuity)?
What is our story or narrative?
What meaningful connection does this create (compassion)?

Meaning as How

How do you do this? How does this work?
What does this cause?
How does this make for coherence (fittingness, makes sense)?

Meaning as So-What

What does this lead to?
So what? What will result from this?

Meaning as Who

Who are you? Who do we become together?
What does this mean for our authenticity or integrity?

Chapter 6

THE QUALITY

OF MEANING

"The state of being without a system of values is psycho-pathogenic...
The human being needs a framework of values, a philosophy of life,
a religion or religion-surrogate to live by and understand by,
in the same sense that he needs sunlight, calcium, or love.
This I have called the 'cognitive need to understand.'"
Abraham Maslow (1968, p. 206)

"In treatment, process is what's important, content is a handmaiden.
Your presence and connection evoke the healing."
Virginia Satir

While the ability to *make* meaning is the human heritage and the human adventure, you cannot make just any meaning. That will not do. Yes, you and the rest of us are a class of life who make meaning and yet if you want to live fully and joyfully *you have to make high quality meaning*—you have to invent, construct, and innovate meanings that are rich, robust, powerful, inspiring, encouraging, vigorous, and life-enhancing.

The reason for this is obvious; meanings come in a wide range of quality. There are lots of meanings that are toxic and dysfunctional. Toxic meanings will sicken your life and diminish you as a person. So just as you can create meanings that are fabulous and inspirational, you can also create meanings that diminish your potentials, that sabotage your highest and best as a person, and that spread thought-virus to others to poison your social life and relationships.

Turning to the subject of the quality of the meanings that you create highlights a basic Neuro-Semantic principle:

> *The quality of the meanings that you make—create and determine the very quality of the life you live.*

Regarding the quality of the meanings that you create and experience, there is a wide range of degrees of quality from low to high. Where meaning is *degraded,* there will be a psychological devastation creating misery and unhappiness, and undermining a person's sense of being a healthy human being.

In fact, reduce, degrade, or rob a human being of meaning and meaningfulness, and the person will sicken, weaken, and suffer the pathologies of meaninglessness. When you are deprived of meaning, no matter how much you have to eat and drink, no matter if you're a multi-millionaire and have fame and influence, *take meaning away* and you can even lose the desire to live. Meaning plays that important a role in your life and well-being. What are the different qualities of meanings that we humans can create?

Meaning Scale
So let's begin by scaling meaning as depicted in *Figure 6:1.* Obviously there are different levels of quality of meanings that you can construct, we can now create a *Meaning Scale* and begin to gauge *the quality of meaning* on a continuum. In the following diagram, I have created such a continuum and have turned it upright as a vertical scale. This enables you to now gauge the quality of the meanings that you create and live by from 0 to 10. This gives you the ability to evaluate and distinguish different qualities of meaning and to choose high quality meanings over low quality ones.

Figure 6:1

Meaning Scale and Index

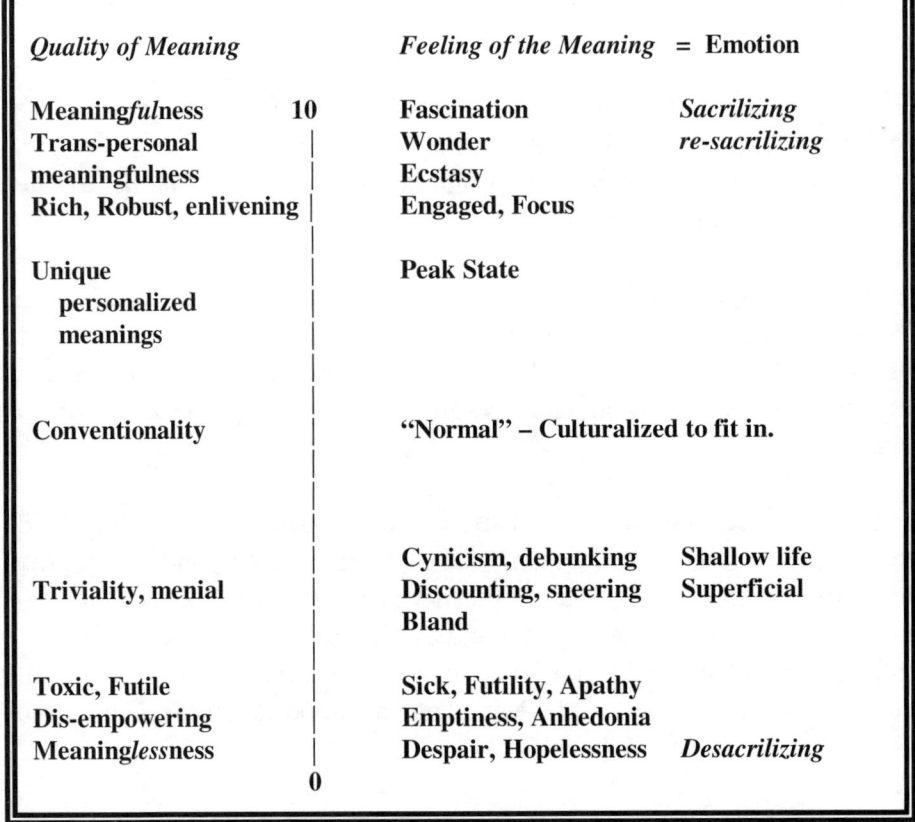

Quality of Meaning		*Feeling of the Meaning*	= **Emotion**
Meaning*ful*ness	**10**	**Fascination**	*Sacrilizing*
Trans-personal		**Wonder**	*re-sacrilizing*
meaningfulness		**Ecstasy**	
Rich, Robust, enlivening		**Engaged, Focus**	
Unique		**Peak State**	
personalized			
meanings			
Conventionality		**"Normal" – Culturalized to fit in.**	
		Cynicism, debunking	**Shallow life**
Triviality, menial		**Discounting, sneering**	**Superficial**
		Bland	
Toxic, Futile		**Sick, Futility, Apathy**	
Dis-empowering		**Emptiness, Anhedonia**	
Meaning*less*ness		**Despair, Hopelessness**	*Desacrilizing*
	0		

I have designed this meaning scale so that 0 stands for meanings that are *meaningless* and at the other end, 10 stands for those that are *meaningful*. Between these polar extremes we can locate futile (0-2), trivial and superficial meanings (3 to 4), conventional meanings relative to the culture and environment you live in (5 to 6), individually unique meanings that excite and give a sense of direction to life (7 to 8), then finally the most highly meaningful meanings that are sacred and expansive as you live for, and contribute to something, bigger than yourself (9-10).

In *Figure 6:1* you can also see that given the quality of the meaning that you attribute to something, there is a corresponding emotional state that you will experience. That is, the quality of the meanings that you create simultaneously

> *The quality of the meanings that you make—create and determine the very quality of the life you live.*

generates the quality and content of your emotional life.   This is critical. You can have no higher or better emotional quality of life than the quality of the meanings that you cognitively construct. These two facets of human experience go hand-in-hand.

Given this, we might say that "meaning is our daily food!" This corresponds to what Jesus said in his classic statement, "Man does not live by bread alone." We have to have more. Of course, we do live by bread at the basic or primary level. Abraham Maslow said that we "only live by bread alone" when we do *not* have any bread. So one of the first meanings in life relates to our basic needs for surviving. Yet even then, as Frankl noted, even at the lowest and barely survival levels of life as in a concentration camp, *man lives by meaning*. Meaningfulness in life is what feeds us, is what nourishes our souls.

Quality Controlling Meanings
If the quality of your meanings is the quality of your state, the quality of your emotions, you can gauge the quality of your life by running a *quality control* on your meanings. Do this to make sure that you have high quality meanings as the frames for your self and your life. We have to do that because there is no inherent quality control process within your neurology.

With regard to what you put into your mouth and process via digestion does have a "quality control" process. You have within your brain-digestion system a process whereby if something is noxious and making you sick, you can vomit. You can expel it before it poisons you and undermines your overall well-being. But your mind doesn't have any automatic instinctive way of doing that. Mentally, your brain simply processes whatever you put into it. Hence, the old computer motto: "GIGO: Garage in; Garage out."

If you put toxic, crazy, hurtful, ugly, and dysfunctional ideas and beliefs into your mind, your mind-body system will simply process that information and then seek to actualize it. There's no automatic *quality control* for your mind. For that, you have to set some criteria and standards. You have to consciously decide what fits and what does not for your life. And that means to rise up to this level and "run a quality control" on your meanings. This also represents one of the central ways that you take charge of your meanings—emotions—life.

> Maslow (1968, p. 153)
> "The neurotic is not emotionally sick, he is cognitively wrong!"

Quality Controlling Cognitive Distortions

If you want a way to diminish the quality of your meanings and therefore life, adopt any one of a dozen or more cognitive distortions. Then you will have the power to make yourself and others miserable.

What are cognitive distortions?

> They are *the thinking patterns* that you first used as you constructed meaning as a child. They are the distortions that ultimately disempower by creating limitations. For an adult, a cognitive distortion is *a style of thinking and processing information* that distorts things in a non-useful way.[1]

These thinking styles or patterns are mostly *the primitive ways of thinking* which you learned as a child and if you perpetuate today will compose faulty perceptions and increase your misery. Yet when you use these ways of thinking and reasoning as an adult, you inevitably create ill-formed and inaccurate mental models that imprison you in non-sense and limiting possibilities. These make up your meaning attribution and explanatory styles. And because everything habituates, repeat them and they will become your unconscious patterns for processing information— your automatic frames.

Figure 6:2 **List of Cognitive Distortions** 1. Over-generalizing 2. All-or-nothing thinking (Dichotomizing) 3. Labeling 4. Blaming 5. Mind-reading 6. Prophesying 7. Emotionalizing 8. Personalizing 9. Awfulizing 10. Should-ing 11. Filtering 12. Impossibility thinking 13. Discounting	**Figure 6:3** **List of Empowering Cognitions** 1. Contextual thinking 2. Both-and-thinking 3. Reality-testing 4. Responsibility thinking 5. Current sensory information 6. Tentative predictive thinking 7. Witness thinking 8. Objective thinking 9. Meta-cognitive thinking 10. Choice thinking 11. Perspective thinking 12. Possibility thinking 13. Appreciative thinking

The solution to this dilemma is actually simple: *Recognize them.* This is a great first step to clarity and choice. Unrecognized cognitive distortions actually set up what we call "buttons" so that certain things can *get* you and "push your buttons." When that happens, you then *react* in unthinking and defensive ways thereby giving power to others to rattle your cage.[2]

Quality controlling your meaning-making at this level means stepping back from your thinking itself, from your style and pattern of constructing meaning and looking at it rather then the content of your thoughts.

- How cloudy and unclean (distorted) is your creation of meanings?
- Could the problem be your style and pattern rather than the content of your thinking?

Its an undeniable fact: *You have a fallible brain.* Fallible means that it is "liable to error." It easily and often makes mistakes. Yet if you are making mistakes and generating basic errors about things at a meta-level of processing, then your cognitive distortions actually provide you a powerful leverage point for transformation.

> There's no automatic *quality control* for your mind. For that, you have to set some criteria and standards.

After all, these are the patterns by which you *explain* things and *make sense* of things. When this happens, your very way of making meaning can itself becomes sick and dis-empowering.

Given the understanding about cognitive thinking patterns, the problem that people experience does not just exist at *the content level, but at the process level.* Consider this the statement: "I'll never be a success; everything I do fails; I am just such a big failure!" The problem here is not only this thought, even more so it is the *kind of thinking* that generates it: all-or-nothing thinking, over-generalizing, personalizing, awfulizing. The real problem is the *thinking / processing frames* even more than the specific painful thoughts.

That's why you can change the content of these thoughts, but if that way of thinking, information processing, and meaning-construction has not been identified and addressed, you have only dealt with one specific symptomatic response, not the problem itself. *The problem is the interpretative frames.* So quality controlling these hidden frames that lurk in the background and which are typically invisible to awareness, is the real solution—a meta solution. This is the place where you can leverage the whole system of your thinking-and-experiencing and facilitate an unleashing from that way of meaning-making.

In *Figure 6:2* I have provided a list of the classic cognitive distortions as generated by Albert Ellis and Aaron Beck in the field of Cognitive Psychology. These thinking patterns are fabulous ways to make yourself and others miserable if that's what you want to do.[1] By way of contrast, *Figure 6:3* offers a list of thinking styles that are richer and more accurate. Since this is such a critical aspect of meaning-making, I have included an extensive description of the cognitive distortions at the end of this chapter. This will allow you to familiarize yourself with them and practice identifying them and updating them with the empowering cognitions.

We regularly practice and use this awareness of cognitive distortions in Neuro-Semantics. We use them as a *checklist* so that we can clean up the hidden processing frames that create unresourceful "dragon" states and that keeps a traumatizing process in place.[3]

Quantity and Quality for Semantically Loading

Semantically loading is a phrase that we use in Neuro-Semantics when we want to speak about *the amount of, or quantity of, meaning that a person invests in something.* So when we ask, "How much meaning have you invested in this idea, person, experience, etc.?" we are asking about the quantity of meaning. This is also true when we ask, "How intense is this for you?" That's because the more meaning that you invest in something, the more it means to you, the more you will feel it, the more it will drive you, the more energy it will produce, and the more it will govern your thinking, perceiving, valuing, etc.

- How much meaning have you attributed to your past experience with that person?
- How much meaning do you attribute to your past?
- How much meaning do you give to food, to eating, to eating out and socializing?

Name your subject and ask these questions. Whatever the answer, it speaks about how *semantically loaded* that thought, concept, person, or experience is for you. Is it highly loaded or is it just barely loaded with meaning? Does it need more meaning? Does it need less?

To semantically load is to give lots of meaning and highly significant meanings to something. It is to layer multiple meanings so that an event, person, or experience now comes to be seen and felt as highly meaningful. It is to *sacralize*—to view something as ultimately valuable or valuable in and of itself. Yet not everything is inherently valuable. That's why not all sacralizing is useful or beneficial. If you give too much meaning to something which cannot bear it, you will treat it as far more important than it is and thereby distort its importance.

Conversely, we often fail to semantically load an experience, idea, concept, etc. with enough meaning. It is *just* whatever it is and not semantically significant enough to provide the drive, the passion, and the motivation that you need. Take exercise. "It is *just* exercise." So, how much meaning do you invest in exercise? Very much? Or is the problem with getting yourself to exercise the very fact that it means so little to you?

Now around the world, most people have given far too much meaning to food and to eating. And during the holidays, people give even more meanings to food. And so, surprise, surprise! People are over-eating even to the point of becoming obese. They don't over-eat to get fat. They don't over-eat to ruin their health. They over-eat because they have a belief frame about food that semantically loads eating so that holding back and refusing to eat seems like, and feels like, such painful experiences self-denial, asceticism, and even starvation. That's why most of us *psycho-eat*. We eat for purposes other than health, energy, and vitality. Most of us eat for love, reward, de-stressing, the good life, being social, following the customs, etc. When we do so, our eating is semantically loaded.

Because, as a meaning-maker, you are always giving meaning to things, asking about the *quantity or intensity* of your meaning enables you to discover if you have invested enough or too much meaning. Knowing that, then you can adjust the amount of meaning that you have attributed. Yet beyond the amount of quantity, you can also look at meaning in terms of *quality*. Ths gives yet another set of questions:
- What is the quality of the meanings that you have invested in X?
- Is the quality of the meaning poor, low, rich, robust, or delightful?
- Is the quality of the meaning you give to X rich and robust enough when you navigate that experience?
- Do you feel that something is meaningless, futile, or trivial?

Sometimes the problem with exercising having such low meaning and needing to be more semantically loaded isn't about the quantity of meaning, but the quality. Given that we can now ask:
"What would be the richest and most exciting meaning you could

give to exercising?"

"What meaning could you invent that you would find inspiring?"

If I asked you these questions, would you be able to immediately pop out five to ten really great answers? Or would you stutter? Would you be stopped in your steps? Would my questions leave you feeling blank? Sometimes we just have not thought long enough and thoroughly enough to give something the abundance of meanings that it needs to be felt motivating. Sometimes we have just not explored the possibilities of great meanings that would make an experience more life-enhancing. And if you have not done that, then no wonder you have not meta-stated the experience with more meanings.

What is the quality of your meanings about food? If you load it up with a lot of rich psychological meanings like "good life," "reward," "love," etc., not only is there a lot of meaning, but the meanings are also rich, significant, expansive, even transcendental. Do this and you will be essentially trying to self-actualize through food! But, of course, in the long run that will not work. Food isn't designed for that. Yet because that's the attributed meaning you've given to food, no wonder you find the experience of eating so semantically loaded. You have loaded it with both high quantity and quality of meanings.

How can you tell if something is semantically loaded for yourself or another person? First there will be a lot of emotion with it. As a person talks about the experience or idea, he or she will be animated. Perhaps even passionate! And whether the animation is positive or negative, the key is the energy in the person's body, voice, eyes, etc. That's because *emotion is how you feel meaning*. Meaning shows up in our bodies as emotions. So where there is emotion, where there is a "button" that can be pushed that "gets" us, there is meaning and semantic loadedness.

And there are other signs. Look for what the person stresses or emphasizes in language: listen for embedded words, commands, questions, and statements.[4] These typically indicate that the person has semantically loaded those particular words. Observe also patterns—actions, gestures, words, etc. These are repeated several times typically indicate that something is semantically loaded. Repetition of repeated behaviors (patterns) indicate the loading of meaning.

Sacralizing— The Ultimate in Making Quality Meanings
If you really want to make some wonderful meanings of high quality, learn how to sacralize. And what is sacralizing?

> *Sacralizing* refers to the ability to see a person or event "under the aspect of eternity," to see things as precious, sacred, special, highly significant and important.

Maslow wrote about sacralizing and exploring it and in doing so said:

> "This is the most important way of helping a person move toward self-actualization."

Sacralizing involves a fresh appreciation for all of life. It is the ability to look at things with a naiveness and newness. And with that perspective then you avoid the toxic problem of getting used to your blessings. A freshness of appreciations means you are able to savor the qualities of an experience. Maslow speaks about this in these words:

> "I have become convinced that getting used to our blessings is one of the most important non-evil generators of human evil, tragedy, and suffering." (1970, p. 163)

Ultimately sacrilizing means choosing to always give rich meanings to things. Anyone can think positively when things are going well, to think positively when things are not going well, that is the real test of optimism and your ability to sacralize.

> "The creativeness of the self-actualized man seems rather to be kin to the naive and universal creativeness of unspoiled children. A fundamental characteristic of human nature— a potentiality given to all human beings at birth." (1970, 170-171)

Now a paradox emerges with this ability. Now you can even make the basic needs sacred through integrative thinking: both profane *and* sacred at the same time.

> "People who enjoy and are committed to the B-Values also enjoy their basic need-gratifications more because they make them sacred.

... to live the spiritual life, you don't have to sit on top of a pillar for ten years. Being able to live in the B-Values somehow makes the body and all its appetites holy." (1971:187, B-value stands for *Being*-value, the meta-values of self-actualization.)

Sacralizing includes an openness to fun, enjoyment, and humor. It means operating perspectively from a non-hostile, philosophical humor.

> "The humor of the real consists in large part in poking fun at human beings in general when they are foolish, or forget their place in the universe, or try to be big when they are actually small." (1970, 169)
> "The healthy person [has] a healthy childlikeness ... the most mature human beings are also childlike. ... the most mature people are the ones that can have the most fun." (1971:89). They can regress at will.
> "A truly integrated person can be both secondary and primary; both childish and mature. He can regress and then come back to reality, becoming then more controlled and critical in his responses." (1971:90)

Sacralizing as an openness to awe and mystery facilitates the peak experiences of self-actualization where there is wonder, loss of self, self-forgetfulness as the awesome over-whelms you with the sense the enormity of the experience. Maslow wrote about Aldous Huxley in this regard:

> "He was perpetually marveling at how interesting and fascinating everything was, by wondering like a youngster at how miraculous things are, by saying frequently, 'Extraordinary! Extraordinary!' He could look out at the world with wide eyes, with unabashed innocence, awe, and fascination..." (1971: 38)

*Emotion is how you **feel** meaning.* Meaning shows up in our bodies as emotions.

Sacralizing is a loving response to life and to others.

> "We *must* understand love; we must be able to teach it, to create it, to predict it, or else the world is lost to hostility and to suspicion." (1970, 181)
> "Love actualizes potentials."   "Not only does love perceive

potentialities but it also actualizes them. The absence of love certainly stifles potentialities and even kills them. Personal growth demands courage, self-confidence, even daring; and non-love from the parent or the mate produces the opposite, self-doubt, anxiety, feelings of worthlessness and expectations of ridicule, all inhibitors of growth and of self-actualization." (1968, p. 98)

Love is an admiration and awe of the beauty of life and values. It asks for nothing, it is an extending of yourself for the growth, well-being of another without expectations of return.

"We can enjoy a painting without wanting to own it, a rosebush without wanting to pluck from it, a pretty baby without wanting to kidnap it, a bird without wanting to cage it, and so also can one person admire and enjoy another in a non-doing or non-getting way." (1970, 197)

Neuro-Semantic Learnings for a Neuro-Semanticist

Meaning is not enough, it has to be quality meaning as well as the quality of your meaning-making. In this chapter, did you learn several things that will powerfully and profoundly enrich the quality of your meanings and enable you to step up to the highest levels of meaningfulness?

1) Take time to go through the dimensions of your life (work, family, hobby, health, fitness, spiritual, economical, career, etc.) and identify where you are on *the quality scale* of the meanings you give to each of these areas.

2) What cognitive distortions do you habitually fall back on which lower the quality of your meanings? Will you take time this week and in the weeks to come to run some *checks* on the quality of your meaning-making? Make a copy of the list of the Cognitive Distortions and take it with you so you can use it as a checklist for your thinking and conversations, especially when you become stressed.

3) At what level of flexibility in creating a wide-range of meanings do you live? What is your next level for expanding your meaning-making?

Meta-States   Conceptual: Cognitive Unconscious

Primary State   Primary Consciousness

Embodied   Embodied Consciousness
                                         Neural Unconsciousness

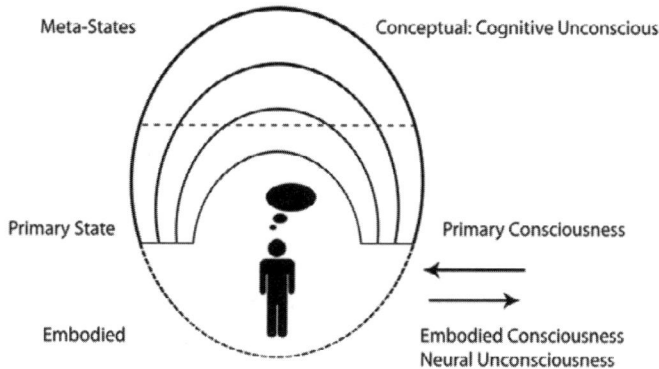

Cognitive Distortions

1. Generalizing; over-generalizing; Jumping to Conclusions; Making Pervasive.

> Taking only a few facts, or none at all, jumping to premature conclusions, and assuming them to be true. Assuming that a negative experience in one area pervades every aspect of life. This creates false cause-effect structures.

2. Judging; judgments, Evaluating.

> Jumping from sensory-based facts to evaluations and judgments without awareness of doing so, then assuming that your evaluations are just the facts.

3. All-or-nothing thinking—Making things pervasive; universal quantifiers.

> Polarizing at extremes, hence, black-or-white thinking. Either-or thinking positing options as two-valued choices, either this or that.
>> Gives no other choices, nothing in the middle; Aristotle's excluded middle.

4. Labeling; Nominalizing; Name Calling.

> Assuming that a name or label can accurately and adequately

describe something. Labeling over-generalizes to reduce reality to just a word, confusing a verbal map with the territory.

5. Thingify-ing; Event Thinking, Elementalism.
Viewing things as separate events, elements. Thinking in a linear way from one event to the next event. Viewing reality as comprised of elements, separate parts; event mentality.

6. Identifying — Identifications.
Treating two things as if *the same* and so the confusing of levels. Using the "to be" verb to create identifications: "He is," "she is," "they are." Confuse behavior, role, and experience with self.

7. Over-Simplifying.
Viewing the world in linear way as events or elements that over-simplifies things. Want easy and quick fixes, seduced by symptoms for symptomatic solutions.

8. Discounting — Perfectionism, Minimizing thinking.
The mental attitude of rejecting and/or putting down by dis-qualifying possible solutions, successes, or possibilities (as in, "That doesn't count," "That's nothing."). "It could have been better."

9. Mind-reading.
Projecting thoughts, feelings, intuitions onto others without checking your guesses with the person, over-trusting your "intuitions" about other people and seeing them through the lens of your mental filters rather than checking out your interpretations and assumptions.

11. Prophesying; mind-reading the future.
Making things Permanent. Projecting negative outcomes into the future without seeing alternatives or possible ways to proactively intervene. Seeing problems and hurts as permanent, and never-ending.

12. Filtering Out; Deletion.
Over-focusing on one facet of something to the exclusive of

everything else to create a tunnel vision perspective. Filtering out what's positive and solutions.

13. Blaming; defensive thinking.

Accusatory thinking that transfers blame and responsibility for a problem to someone or something else. Fear and/or refusal to be wrong in your eyes and the eyes of others.

14. Emotionalizing; wishful thinking; reactive thinking.

Complex Equivalence: emoting is cognition. Taking counsel of your emotions as an infallible source for reality, assuming that if feeling an emotion makes it must real and that you must act on that feeling. "If I want something, I should have it." "My wishing will make it real." "I have to feel it to do it."

15. Personalizing; Identification.

Perceiving circumstances and actions of others as targeted toward yourself, perceiving world through the ego-centric filter that everything, or most things, is about yourself. Ego-centric thinking.

16. Awfulizing; Pseudo-Words.

Emotionalizing + Labeling = Awfulizing. Imagining the worst possible scenario and amplifying it and calling it "Awful" ("This is awful!") without any clear indication about what *awful* actually refers to. Spread an unpleasant event to other experiences, making it pervasive.

17. Should-ing; Demandingness; Modal Operators.

Using the words "should" or "must" to pressure yourself and others to conform to rules. When using "must," we are "musterbating" (Ellis).

"The tyranny of the shoulds" (Horney).

18. Can't-ing; Taboo-ing; Modal Operator.

Imposing semantic limits on yourself and others using the word "can't" which presupposes that there is some law or rule that constrains us from doing something.

Problems that Sabotage Solutions for an Empowering Response

1. Generalizing; over-generalizing.
Limits finer distinctions
Hides critical success factors.
Blinds to possibilities for solution

Jumping to Contextual thinking.
Inquire about the context of the information and index by asking: what, when, where, which, who, and why? Ask about vague terms and unspecified nouns and verbs.
Outcome: clarity and precision.

2. Judging; judgments, Evaluating.

Blinds you to the actual facts.
Creates confusion of levels; leads to fights and arguments about so-called "facts." Blinds you from seeing how you contribute to arguments.

Description; sensory-based thinking.
Distinguishes between the sensory and evaluative levels, restores proper role of facts, enables critical distinctions.

3. All-or-nothing thinking —
Making things pervasive.
Universal Quantifiers
Eliminates and hides all values in between the polar choices.

Both-and Thinking: In-between thinking.
Test situation to see if there is some option in-between the extremes. To what degree?

Sets up extremes as in manic-depression.
Undermines creativity and choices.
Creates obsessions, compulsions.

Gauge for percentages, scale from 0 to 10.
Check contexts.
Outcome: expands choice.

4. Labeling; Nominalizing; Name Calling.
Sells a person short by putting into

a box and assuming that's all the person is.
Hides reality in a label.

Map-Territory and Reality-testing thinking.
          Ask: Is this just a label, just a word?
Explore: In what way is it bad, undesirable?
What are you referring to? When? Where?
Under what conditions?
Outcome: more accurate mapping.

5. Thingify-ing; Event Thinking,
Elementalism; over-simplifies reality;
fails to make critical distinctions.

Process thinking, developmental thinking;
De-Nominalizing.
Looking for and thinking in terms of

patterns of change; seeing the slow, gradual processes. Thinking systemically about experiences.

6. Identifying — Identifications.
Confuses things, fails to make distinctions, limits self-definition

to identifications.

E-prime / Process thinking.
Challenge and replace "to be" verbs with verbs that actually describe what a person is

doing. *Not: "I am a father" but "I father..."*

7. Over-Simplifying.
Blinds to the complexity of the world. Feeds impatience and undermines persistence.

Systems thinking.
Views world and experiences in terms of systems complexity, seeking leverages for effective changes.

8. Discounting — Perfectionism.
Minimizing thinking.
Limits small approximates of success and solutions from being recognized and developed.

Appreciative thinking.
Ask: What counts for you? In what way? How can this be valued? For what? What else? Do you have permission to make mistakes?
Outcome: Reinforce small steps, enrich sense of value, awaken appreciation.

9. Mind-reading.
Limits seeing and dealing with a person based on facts of sensory data.

Projects beliefs onto others.
Confuses self and others.

Sensory thinking.
What are the facts? See-hear-feel facts? Ask: How do you know that? How draw that conclusion? What are the probabilities?
What are you feeling or thinking?
Outcome: straightens out relationship, encourages dialogue, keep things present.

14. Emotionalizing; wishful thinking; reactive thinking.
Limits hope, belief, vision, dreaming, possibilities.
Makes problems permanent and so

Observational / Witnessing thinking.
Study trends, factors, and causes that contribute to an experience. Study consequences and probabilities.
       Outcome: Opens future, identifies
       leverage

eliminates solutions.

points, increase ability to influence.

12. Filtering Out; Deletion.
Limits full perspective.
Blinds one from seeing beyond the

tunnel vision.

Perspective / meta-cognitive thinking.
Step back and identify filters that create
tunnel vision. Take third-person
perspective
to empathize with another's view
Outcome: expands awareness to see other
perspectives.

13. Blaming; defensive thinking.
Limits recognizing response-ability.

Wastes energy accusing someone.
Blinds one to responses for change.
Impairs power of responsibility.

Responsibility / Denominalizing / systemic
thinking. Ask: what am I response-able
for?
To whom? Is this a response that others
make? Question the *nominalization*, What
is the process? The action? What action
has been "named" (nominalized)? What is
the system? Who is in it? How does the
system work?
Outcome: Clarity, see processes rather
than things.

14. Emotionalizing; wishful thinking;
reactive thinking. Limits choice by
creating an emotional determinism.

Impairs healthy use of emotions.
Creates a dependency on emotions.
Semantically overloads emotions
with too much meaning.

Observational / Witnessing thinking.
Step back and just observe. Witness senses,
facts, activities without making
any judgment.
Suspend evaluation; witness what *is.*
Outcome: increases choices and options,
stops the coloring of things by emotions,
obtain cleaner information.

15. Personalizing; Identification.
Limits clear perceptions.
Blinds one to seeing world through

one's ego filters.

Objective, observing thinking.
Step back and take second or third
perceptual position; What does
this look like
from neutral observer? Could this be about
the source rather than me?
Outcome: make things more objective, gain
clean information, distinguish self and
world.

16. Awfulizing; Pseudo-Words.
Limits problem-solving skills.
Prevents you from working on
creative solutions.

Misdirects energy to whining and
complaining.

Meta-cognitive thinking.
Ask about patterns and structures above and
beyond the story and content. Identify
thinking patterns. Question words and
terms
for what they refer to.
Outcome: Expand awareness of factors in
the back of the mind, see and identify
patterns and leverage points of change.

17. Should-ing; Demandingness;
Modal Operators.
Limits a sense of choice.

Leashes you to a sense of dreadful
duty. Eliminates sense of choice.

Choice thinking.

Test "should," "must," and "have to."
Why?
Who says? What is the rule? What is the
demand? Change to "want" or "prefer."
Outcome: prevents addiction and build up
off pressure. Keeps wants and desires
healthy.

18. Can't-ing; Taboo-ing;
Modal Operator.
Limits ideas about what's possible.

Stunts ideas of human potential
Impairs ability to dream and to take
risks.

Possibility thinking.

      Test "can'ts." Is physical or
      psychological
"can't?" Ask: What stops you? "Do you
have permission? "What would it look,
sound or feel like?"
Outcome: Frees from constraints and opens
up new possibilities.

CLEANING UP THE DISTORTIONS

When you are "cognitively wrong" (Maslow) your perceptions are foggy rather than clean. Mental and emotional pain arises not because we are emotionally sick, but because you are cognitively wrong. You are simply operating from a mistaken map. You have maps that simply do not enable you to navigate the territory very well. You have frames that build an unstable structure and foundation. You have not outgrown the childish thinking patterns that distort and leash your potentials. Every cognitive distortion that governs your perceptions creates misery and undermines your pathway to self-actualization. These cognitive distortions are based on deficiency-cognitions, rather than the *Being*-cognitions that inevitably facilitate self-actualization.

The Pattern:
1) Identify an activity.
> Think of some activity where you are not getting the results that you want.
> What is it? How do you describe it?
> What is your story?

2) List and identify cognitive distortions that create difficulties or limitations.
> Use the cognitive distortions as a check-list. What are the 3 big ones for you?
> Have you specified all of the ones that create problems and difficulties for you or another person?
> Which one do you want to work on right now?

3) Validate and confirm the cognitive distortion.
> Reflect it back to the person.
>> "It sounds like you are thinking about this using *Awfulizing*. As you step back from it, does it seem accurate?"
> How else would you characterize this pattern of thought?

4) Invite the person to a meta-position.
> Does this pattern of thinking reflect one that you typically or often use?
> How long have you used this cognitive distortion in sorting through things?
> Has it served you well? In what way?
> In what way may it have undermined your sense of well-being and accurate processing?
> What more useful way of processing this information would you like to use?

5) Meta-state the distortion to reduce its influence.
> What would you best like to do to reduce its power?
> Would you like to challenge, dispute, and argue against Personalizing, Awfulizing, Should-ing, etc.?
> Are you ready to identify and release these cognitive patterns?

What else will bring these patterns into the light where you can deal with them? What else will break their power of working outside of consciousness? [Journaling, appointing someone as a detector, etc.]

6) *Update the cognitive distortions with empowering thinking patterns.*

As you use the check list of the more enhancing ways of thinking, which one will you use to replace the misery-producing thinking pattern?

Meta-Stating a Resource State

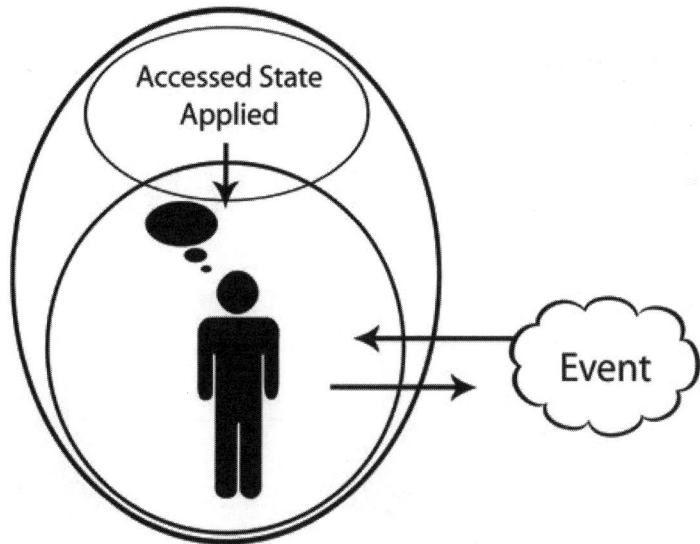

End of the Chapter Notes
1. The Cognitive Distortions came from Albert Ellis and Aaron Beck. For a fuller description of the cognitive distortions and how these founders of Cognitive Psychology used them, see their works, especially, Ellis' *Guide to Rational Living.*

2. When commonly speak about "getting our buttons pushed" we are referring to some stimulus (a word, gesture, facial expression, action, etc.) that we have given lots of meaning to, usually a personal meaning. The result is that we have a *semantic reaction.*

3. A "dragon" state is an unresourceful state, typically because we have turned thoughts and emotions against ourselves, see *Dragon Slaying* (1995, 2000).

4. An *embedded* command or question is also a hypnotic language pattern. It refers to how we can create a sentence within a sentence so that a command or question is embedded inside it. This was modeled from Milton Erickson, see *Patterns of the Hypnotic Techniques of Milton H. Erickson, M.D. Volume I.*

Chapter 7

THE FLEXIBILITY

OF MEANING-MAKING

"Behaving as if meaning were stable
seems to be useful in day-to-day life,
this is how we normally behave."
Steve de Shazer (1991, p. 70)

T he quality of your meaning-making is dependent on a particular facet
of meaning— *your range of flexibility.* That is, your ability to create,
recreate, and change your meanings so you are not stuck or limited by
your current meanings. The less flexibility you have, the more rigid and
stuck you will be with your ideas, your maps about things, and your
subsequent emotions. As a result, less flexibility with meaning will make
you less able to move around conceptually in your meaning-construction.
In that case, your meanings *have* you instead of you *having* your meanings.

The flexibility you have, or don't have, as a meaning-maker then is another
critical distinction about meaning. It supplements the several critical facets
of meaning already explored: *the dimensions, the kinds, the levels, and the
quality* of meaning. It is your flexibility, and the range of your flexibility to
make multiple numbers of meanings regarding anything, that empowers you

with an authentic sense of choice. With that comes the sense that you are truly a meaning-*maker—a creator of the meanings* that comprise the fabric of your life.

∞-Valued Semantics

When Alfred Korzybski analyzed meaning in terms of flexibility, he called for *an ∞-valued (infinite-valued) semantics.* Given that the symbol ∞ is the symbol for infinity and refers to something without an end, an infinite-valued semantics refers to expanding your flexibility in meaning-making so that you are not limited to the one-valued, two-valued, or three-valued semantics.

"Okay, and why is this important?" Because as a semantic class of life, *meaning* is your creation and can therefore be ∞-valued. That is, always being able to create more and more possible meanings for what something means expands your powers for creating more choices in any context. Then you will know at a deep level that there are ∞-valued degrees of conditionality in any word or event.

When it comes to the creation of meaning, every level of your semantics leads to certain *semantic reactions* (SR). It is inevitable. If you invent meaning, and then embody it so that it affects your feelings, your emotions, and your responses, then those responses will be *semantic* responses. Korzybski wrote about how semantic responses can become habituated so that you lose awareness of them and they become your semantic reactions:

> "In human regression or undevelopment, human symbols have degenerated to the values of signals effective with animals, the main difference being in the *degree* of conditionality." (p. 338).
> "Consciousness of abstracting produces *complete conditionality* in our conditional higher order reactions, and so must be the foundation on which a science of man or a theory of sanity and progress, must be built." (p. 339)
> "The ∞-valued semantics is the most general and includes the one-, two-, etc. and few-valued semantics as particular cases. The one-valued semantics of literal identifications are found only among animals, primitive people, infants, and the 'mentally' ill, although more or less serious traces of some identification are found in practically all of us, because these are embodied in the structure of

our language..." (p. 461)

The degree of conditionality in something affects how much choice you actually have as you respond. This corresponds to the NLP template about choice:

> If you have one choice, you are a slave. If you have two choices, you are on the horns of a dilemma. It is only when you have three or more choices that you have true choice.

It is your conscious flexibility in generating meanings—lot of them— that enables you to have true choice in terms of the meaning you give to any given thing, person, or experience. This raises the question of quantity: *How many meanings are you able to generate?* It is the flexibility question par excellence: How flexible are you in shifting your meanings? To only have one choice, "X means Y" is to have no flexibility at all, but to be conditioned for only one response. One mental-emotional response which allows only one behavioral response. This is the world that animals live in. It is also the world of fanatics who have become "true believers" in the absolutism of some creed. Here the person's map *is* the territory. Here a person speaks in absolute terms that closes the possibility of it meaning anything else. "He is a jerk."

As you expand that one choice to two, "X means Y or Z" now you are able to enables you to at least have an either-or, black-or-white choice. This moves you into the world of polar choices. And while that gives you a little more choice, it doesn't give you much choice. Now you will find yourself often on the horns of a dilemma. You have excluded the middle area of all the grays. This is the Aristotelian logic of the excluded middle. Now you live in a world of either-or choice: "You are either a success or a failure." "This is either a great idea or worthless." "If you don't love me, you hate me."

Expanding choice further gives you three or more choices and now the question, "Which is the real or best choice." This facilitates the response of combat and debate. This may not seem like an improvement, yet it is.

And why is that so? Because it calls for critical thinking skills whereby you can evaluate something according to specific criteria that you chose. Of these 3 (or 4 or 7 choices), what are the criteria against which you will weigh the choices?

The next level of development also seems like less of an improvement, but again, it truly is. When people first begin to discover that they can give anything multiple meetings, they typically go through the stage of relativism and may even give up the pursuit for truth since they assume that every choice is equal. "Every meaning is equally legitimate." Yet that is just a stage of cognitive and semantic development. It is not the end state. And it certainly is not the most useful.

Finally comes the full conditionality and flexibility of response as you realize that while you can give anything nearly any meaning, you also realize there are better and worse choices. All choices and meanings are *not* equal. Some meanings are brilliant, other meanings are tragic and toxic. So with awareness of your flexibility and choices, you can set conditions—values, criteria, standards by which you make your choices about the best meanings in a given context.

In the following figure (Figure 7:1), to read it, start at the bottom with the one-valued semantics and then move up the list. *SR* stands for the *semantic reactions* that result for any given level of meaning.

Figure 7:1
Part I (Read from the bottom upward)

Valued Semantics   Significance and Semantic Reactions (SR)

_____ *The Search for the one True Meaning*_____
     /   \

Few-valued semantics Conflictual meaning since a word or event has three or
more meanings.
SR: Arguments, debates. Search for the one true
meaning, introduction of critical thinking skills to test
and debate which is best.

Two-valued semantics Dichotomous meanings since a word or event has two
meanings, it is either X or Y, a polarized view of life.
SR: Either-or, black-or-white thinking, dualistic,
dichotomous thinking, excludes the middle so that
there are no grays.

One-valued semantics Identification "map *is* territory" meaning, a word or
event has but one and only one meaning, failure to
differentiate, confusion of levels.
SR: Absolutist, finalist, fanatic, animalistic use of
symbols as if signals rather than symbols. Words are
things ("the thinghood of words").

Figure 7:1
Part II
(Read from the bottom up)

Valued Semantics   **Significance and Semantic Reactions (SR)**

∞-valued semantics   Multi-ordinal meanings: "At what level?" "In what
                            dimension?" Flexibility in meanings, choice about the
                            most useful, ecological, highest quality meaning that
                            will serve the situation. Probabilistic meanings, since
                            any word or event has ∞-valued meanings, meanings
                            are determined by context and dimension, are
                            probabilistic, to what extent is this or that particular
                            meaning likely to be useful, true, or productive?

                            SR: Instead of a reaction, a chosen response based on
                            what you think is the most ecological meaning.

**Many-valued   Relativist meaning; every word or event has a great
semantics**   many meanings.

                         SR: Skepticism, if everything is relativistic, there is no
                         true meaning, it means whatever you want it to mean.
                         End of arguments and conflicts, non-commitment as
                         giving up the search for meaning.

_____ *The Search for the one True Meaning*_____
   /   \

Examples of Meaning Flexibility

Steve de Shazer in *Putting Difference to Work* (1991) tells the story of a couple in therapy.

> "A woman and her husband came to therapy because, six weeks earlier, she had suddenly developed an 'insatiable' desire for sex; she had become, in her words, a nymphomaniac. During this six week period, she had felt that she had to have sexual intercourse at least once a day before going to sleep." (p. 63)

The presenting problem that the woman offered to the therapist is one-valued. She defined her problem as being a "nymphomaniac." That was the meaning that she had constructed about what was wrong in her life. But as we know, *the presenting problem* is just that, *what is first presented* and, more often than not, not the real problem. In fact, most often the presenting problem is a symptom of the real problem and a test for the helper. And of course, as a meaning-maker, even the "real" problem is the problem that we create or co-create with a therapist, consultant, or coach. It is what we negotiate via the therapeutic or coaching conversation.

Steve de Shazer describes the conversation that the therapist had with the couple and how the therapist went about looking for exceptions in order to construct a more solvable problem. Then he heard the husband say, "For me, it's more of a sleep problem for both of us." When the therapist heard that, he used that to begin defining the problem as insomnia, a less serious problem, one easier to solve. With that possible frame, the complaint also became undecidable. It could have one of two possible meanings: a sexual disturbance or a sleep disturbance. Which was it? Was it nymphomania or insomnia?

That then led to asking about the bedroom and suddenly there was a third possibility: a bed-as-context problem. Maybe the problem wasn't inside the woman at all, maybe it was something about the bedroom. When the conversation later turned to what was different in the six weeks of the problem, it turned out that the woman had begun to exercise for one hour a day. So maybe this was an exercise problem. Now we had four possibilities of what "the problem" could be.

What did "her desire for sex so she could sleep" really mean? What can we understand about what is causing this disturbance? What can we understand about this?

- It's a sexual disturbance problem: nymphomaniac.
- It's a sleep disturbance problem: insomnia.
- It's an exercise disturbance problem: over-stimulated late at night.
- It's a bedroom design problem: uncomfortable context or bed.

Upon expanding the possible meanings of the woman's case, I love what Steve de Shazer then wrote:

> "At this point in the session, the meaning(s) of what was going on was set adrift in a sea of possible meanings." (de Shazer, p. 66)

Ah ha! He had created a context of ∞-valued semantics. So what happened? As the conversation moved to playing with the label "sleep problem," and since it did not carry the highly pathological meanings that "sexual problem" did, and since the client accepted this new name for her compliant, "the therapist focused the conversation around the difficulties with getting to sleep." The Brief Psychotherapist therefore suggested an intervention using some experiments as the task:

> 1) Quit exercising for now and notice what happens.
> 2) If you are awake for one hour after going to bed, get up and do hateful household chores like oven cleaning (attach aversion to staying awake).
> 3) If you are awake for one hour, continue to lie there but with eyes wide open, concentrating on keeping her tongue from touching the roof of her mouth. (Strain the alertness of being awake to boring somatic distinctions!)

Two weeks later she wrote and said that her "insatiable need for sex" was but "a symptom of her insomnia" and that her "sleep patterns and libido had returned to normal." Interesting.

> "Perhaps the new name, with its attached meanings, was enough to solve the client's problem and the suggestions were unnecessary." (p. 67)

With her one-valued meaning at the beginning of the session, she had a singular problem. It was what it was—it was nymphomania, and that's all it was; so fix it, cure it. Then, by exploring "the problem," it became less solid, more fluid. Now she had an undecidable problem, it could be one of two choices. That now made it two-valued. "This or that." Then as the conversation continued to massage and play with the situation, there were four-choices about what it could be, what it could mean. Now the meaning-construction was completely in flux. And it is this flexibility of meaning-construction that provided the ability to choose the one that could be solved and solved more easily. After all, if it is constructed then why make the solution harder than it need to be?

Negotiating Meaning

Because meanings are constructed—all of our meanings are fluid, tentative, and changeable. This is great! You are not stuck with your meanings. You can

> The *paradox* is that you will be able to facilitate great change if you don't enter to change things.

change them! And given this nature of your semantics, you have some room for negotiating the meaning that you want. Yet how far does this go? Surely, you can't give any meaning to a word or experience. There are some constraints about what something means. A banana is not an organization; a clock is not love. Yet even within these constraints, if you are flexible in your meaning-making skills, you can live by, and practice using an ∞-valued semantics.

What if we applied this to something serious like depression? So what about depression? How could you negotiate a more useful meaning for the phenomenon that we label with the nominalization, "Depression?" What else could it mean when a person complains that he or she feels depressed? If one has symptoms like a vague, inexplicit dissatisfaction, with a sense of emptiness or futility, with decreased desire for food, sex, fun, etc. These are the most common symptoms of depression and are among the key ones used in the Beck Depression Inventory to measure the degree of a person's depression.[1]

After all, trying to solve "depression" is a very big monster to solve. If instead, you meta-model that nominalization ("depression") and ask about what and how a person is depressing, you will then be able to reframe the meaning more productively. So what else could it mean than psychological depression? Perhaps it means—

1) One is suffering through a mid-life crisis and needs a new fresh goal to pursue.

2) One is aging and feeling tired and needs some new activities for some new vitality in life.

3) One is experiencing the lack of healthy foods and exercise.

4) One is unhappy with his job and is feeling a new restlessness for something more challenging.

5) One is unhappy with a marriage that needs to be rejuvenated.

6) One has fulfilled his goals and simply does not have a new goal in place yet.

7) One is experiencing a loss and hasn't directly grieved for it and replaced it with a new value.

It is the fluid–flexible nature of meaning that allows you to expand your semantics so you can operate by ∞-value semantics and create true choice in your life. Doing that is "taking the red pill" and taking ownership of your Matrix of Meanings.

Problem Embracing

The key to opening up meaning lies in how you enter into the semantic reality that someone offers you. Do you enter with respect and honor? Do you create with curiosity and openness? Or do you enter with judgment ready to and impatient to fix the person? Do the latter and you will not be allowed entrance. Do the former and you'll be trusted.

The *paradox* is that you will be able to facilitate great change if you don't enter to change things. The paradox is to enter welcoming, accepting, and embracing whatever someone might call a problem, a complaint, or an excuse. Let your first response be one of entering into the "problem" rather than trying to fix it or make it go away.[2]

After all, what is a problem? It is another construct. It is a mental construct about the gap that exists between your present state and the state that you desire. "Problems" (another nominalization) only occur in the mind, not outside in the external world. As such a problem involves your ideas, desires, hopes, expectations, and anticipations about something that you want to be different. *So even your problems are constructs of meaning that you invent regarding the gap. This means that **you** invent your problems.* And if that's the case, then be sure to invent great ones! That means that *how* you define the problem, state the problem, and describe the problem enables or disables your ability to solve it.[3]

When you have a problem, it is only a problem when *you want something more or different than what you currently have.* So ultimately, problems are human concepts that you and I invent. They do not exist. Not in the outside world! Problems exist in the minds of humans. Problems are called into existence by a person's mental and conceptual understanding and interpretation of things. As such, problems involve meta-frames of beliefs, values, expectations, anticipations, fears, etc.

When you have a problem, you have an interpretative frame about some empirical facts with the result that *what you have* and *what you want* are different. This creates *the gap*—which is the problem that you feel. The

> *Even problems are constructs of meaning— you invent the gap, you invent your problems.* So invent great ones— solvable ones!

empirical facts describe what *is.* How you interpret, explain, and appraise those raw sensory facts calls, or doesn't call, a "problem" into existence.

This means that the person is never the problem; nor is reality ever the problem. *The frame is always and only the problem.* It is the interpretative frame itself that makes a situation or a person "a problem." So, first explore what beliefs or understandings help you frame a given situation as a problem. Then, as a meaning-maker creator, invent solvable problems that will enhance your life.

Problems often hide as the hidden frames within your assumptions and presuppositions. This requires that you step back from a frame and for a meta-reflection as you examine your premises, philosophies, and assumptions that govern your thinking, reasoning, and perceiving. These invisible frames are often the source of problems that seem to arise from nowhere and that may not be solvable.

As an invention of the mind, *a problem is a problem because it means something important to you.* You have given some event, person, or situation certain meanings as you believe something about it. And you dis-value something about the current situation, wanting it to be different. The bottom line: Become a great and powerful problem-designer! Design solvable problems, problems whose solution will make a difference, problems that are fun to solve, problems that will generate lots of money for you, and problems that will activate your highest and best skills to solve.

No wonder that geniuses have written what they have written about problems. Here are some examples of this: John Dewey, for example, said,

"A problem is half-solved if properly stated." And Albert Einstein with Infeild wrote in *The Evolution of Physics*:

> "The formulation of a problem is far more often essential than its solution, which may be merely a matter of mathematical or experimental skills. To raise new questions, new possibilities, to regard old problems from a new angle requires creative imagination and marks real advance in science."

And Abraham Maslow wrote:

> "The best way to view a present problem is to give it all you've got, to study it, and its nature, to perceive *within* it the intrinsic interrelationships, to discover (rather than to invent) the answer to the problem within the problem itself." (p. 61)

> The person is never the problem; nor is reality ever the problem. *The frame is always and only the problem.*

To have great problems and to become a great problem-solver, use your semantic flexibility to generate infinite-value semantics about the "problems" you experience. Ask yourself questions that will expand your choices and gives you the space for moving around in your world:

> How else could I interpret this?
> What other meanings could I give to this, meanings that would empower me and enrich my world?
> What are seven more meanings that I could invent for this?
> What would be the most solvable description of the problem?
> What am I missing? What would be a wild way of explaining this?

The More Meanings— the More Flexibility

The value of having the flexibility to create infinite-valued meanings is that it opens up choices and enables you to frame yourself, others, your work, your world in a way that enriches you, enhances your life, and brings out your best resources. This is the ultimate creativity— to create a multiple list of meanings and to then choose the ones that fit best and that unleash your highest potentials.

Neuro-Semantic Learnings for a Neuro-Semanticist

• Since you invent meaning and since there is tremendous flexibility to the phenomenon of meaning and meaning-making, what something means can be defined along a wide range of things. Knowing this, take something that has low level of meaning in your world and enrich it with ten new meanings.

*   How much flexibility you have in giving meaning to things, in seeing and recognizing that there can be other meanings to something frees you from being a victim of meaning and enables you to become a master of meaning and of your own meaning-making. What triggers negative meanings in you? What new meanings will give you more choice and flexibility?

*   Developing more flexibility in meaning also enables you to have more of a sense of choice when confronted by all other meanings that the media and others seek to impose upon you.

End of Chapter Notes:
1. The Beck Depression Inventory (BDI) has been around since 1980s. You can find it and a full description of it in David Burn's classic book, *The New Mood Therapy*.

2. This is not easily learned. In Module III of Meta-coaching, the *Coaching Mastery* course, we use several patterns to facilitate this: Releasing Judgment, De-Contamination Chamber, and then use 8 days of benchmarking practice to help train out.

3. See the pattern of a Well-Formed Problem in *Games Business Experts Play,* and also the *Unleashing Creativity and Innovation* in the series of Self-Actualization Workshops.

Chapter 8

CULTURES

OF MEANING

"We say 'a touchdown counts six points.' Now, that is not a thought that anyone could have without linguistic symbols. ... why? Because points can exist only relative to a linguistic system for representing and counting points, and thus we can think about points only if we are in possession of the linguistic apparatus necessary for such a system."
John Searle, *The Construct of Social Reality*

Knowledge without context is not knowledge; it's just information.

For any idea, statement, representation, belief, etc. to have meaning, it has to be contextualized. *Context (or reference) is always what enables meaning to emerge.* You experience something as meaningful because of how you understand what *something is* (identification) and your understanding of *how it works* (causation). Doing this frames it in terms of its relationship within and to some context. These kinds of meanings (identity, causation, significance, etc.) require an internal context—first your mental-emotional context of your private thinking and later the external contexts that involve others.

Take, for example, the statement, "How are you?" What does that statement mean? Does not the meaning of that statement depend on its context? The question, "How are you?" in the context of friends is an open inquiry that is equivalent to saying, "Hello, good to see you." Yet in a hospital situation when a doctor asks, "How are you?" that's a very different question and carries a very different meaning. So is the question when a therapist asks it as his opening question for a session. The same question in different contexts signifies different meanings.

> *Context (or reference) is always what enables meaning to emerge.*

In these instances, the meaning of the question changes depending on the context. The contexts controls the meanings. Perhaps we could go further and say, *Without a context, there is no meaning.* And if external contexts play this significant of a role in meaning creation, how much more do internal contexts? Context sets frames by implication and, as such, becomes synonymous with the term "frame."

In speaking about *frames of meaning* I am speaking about the internal contexts that you have in your mind for classifying and understanding things. Your inner contexts operate as your interpretative frames and schemes. To expand this a bit further, it is the context that you use, which you are usually unaware of which creates your meanings. Without those internal frames, you are not able to create meaning. With them, you become a prodigious and prolific meaning-maker.

Cultural Contexts

Here's another factor. When it comes to meaning-making, you are not the only person who constructs meaning, you are not alone in this adventure. In the adventure of meaning-making, *we are all involved.* And when we and others create meanings, each of our meanings are psychological— in our minds and emotions. Yet because they are also in our neurology, we inevitably externalize them so that they can be seen and heard on the outside. And when we humans externalize our meanings, we create "cultures." Meanings externalized become cultural artefacts with real and tangible expressions that can, and do, influence ourselves and others.

This isn't a new phenomenon. Those who came before us created meanings and those before them created meanings and this meaning-making process has been going on for thousands of years. Nor did the meanings that they created end with them, they transferred their meanings to us. That transference of meaning occurs partly in the oral tradition as they taught their children what things mean and what to do with them, and partly in all of the ways they used symbols to hold and communicate those meanings in writings and architecture—books, libraries, art, decorations, media, ritual, ceremonies, education systems, religious systems, etc.

All of this describes what we call *culture.* And while "culture" sounds like a "thing," it is not. Ah, here is another nominalization. Here is another term whose referent we cannot put in a wheelbarrow. "Culture" is not a real noun, it is a nominalization. So what is the hidden verb within this term? As a verb it means "to culture" and "to cultivate." And what do we cultivate? The minds and hearts of our children and everyone else who will receive the cultivation. We cultivate behavior, morals, ethics, attitudes, frames of mind, values, etc.

It is by cultivating our minds and hearts, and those of others, with our meanings that we create the cultures that we then live in. This refers to all of the ways that we have learned to relate to each other—to our rituals, rules, policies, beliefs, values, lifestyles, ways of greeting, celebrating, creating groups, and so on. Because how to be human is not given in our genes or genetic inheritance, we have to learn how to be human. The result of that learning becomes the process of how we cultivate our own minds and hearts and actions, and those of others, to be human in the way we understand and desire to be human. And the content of what we learn becomes the program of the culture that we are then habituated to.

We are *cultural beings* for these reasons. As we grew up and received the particular cultivation via parenting, schooling, religious instruction, etc., we became the cultural person we are today. Nor is this a singular process. We are all multi-cultural.

Being multi-cultural means that each of us do not have just one culture, we have many. There is your family culture in which you grew up, the school culture, business culture, ethnic culture, religious culture, linguistic culture, etc. And where do all of these cultures exist? *In your mind.* And also in the minds of all those who accept a given culture.

Culture is an inside-out phenomenon. It is first created inside as the way you are cultivated to think, emote, speak, act, and relate. Then you

> *Culture is an inside-out phenomenon.*

externalize that culturing. Your culture is then externalized in books, literature, rituals, architecture, music, art, organizations, etc. This formalizes the culture and makes it an external context so that you are continually reminded of it and triggered by it. And it is a living culture as it lives dynamically in you and in the minds-and-hearts of people who accept it, believe in it, and use it as their framework for life. When this happens cultures become *the shared meaning* that lives in the thinking and feeling of a group of people which holds the group together.

Conversely, when a people stop accepting the content of a culture and replace it with other frames of meaning about life and group existence, the old culture dies. It becomes a mere relic of a begone era when people believed and behaved in a certain way. That's why the culture of knights of mediaeval Europe no longer exists. The culture of ancient Egypt of Pharaohs no longer exist. Their architecture continues. Their stories, literature, and even their rituals can continue in movies or ceremonies, but not as a living way of life. So even though cultures generally last longer than the life of a single person, they also can and do die.

The Internalization of Culture
While culture can be and is externalized in so many ways, *culture itself is an internal experience—it is a set of meaning frames in the minds of those who live that culture.* If no one *lives* the cultural frames, we can then say that that culture does not exist. That explains how and why cultures come and go, why a culture can be under attack, why it can be changed, improved, and even designed.

Actually, culture is one of the "logical levels" in your mind. It is a logical level of meanings, beliefs, values, understandings, permissions, prohibitions, identifications, and so on. And unlike most of your frames which you personally construct, your cultural frames are for the most part, frames that you receive through osmosis. You are born into various cultural frames and so you just accept them as "the way things are." And because you are born into various cultures, you tend to accept them from the very beginning. This explains why these frames are mostly unconscious and unquestioned. They make up your most unconscious assumptions and therefore your blind spots.

Interestingly, that which primarily brings these frames into your awareness is the experience of encountering another culture. It is by stepping out of your culture and into another one that most shockingly can make you aware of your own culture. You are then enabled to see it for what it is—perhaps to see it as if for the first time as your culture.

Constructivist-and-Developmentalist theorist Robert Kegan (1994) says that while we make sense of things,

> Where do cultures exist? *In your mind.* And in the minds of all those who accept a given culture. Culture in an inside-out phenomenon.

> "... we do not always take responsibility for it as made. We are more likely to believe that it is 'the way the world is made' (and to leave out the agent of that passively constructed sentence). Some of our meaning-making is completely idiosyncratic and falls under no governance or regularity other than the regularity of our unique personalities. And some of our meaning-making may derive from our membership in various subgroups of the human family, such as social class, ethnicity, gender, and culture. These subgroups may endow us with their own meaning-regulative principles, ways we know or see that derive from our membership in these subgroups." (p. 206)

Most of the cultural meanings that we inherit are those that were already *made* by the people who preceded us. We inherit these meanings as the heritage and richness of the environment in which we are reared. As creatures of our cultures we learn these meanings by osmosis, meanings that inform us of what's important and what's not, what to eat, how to create people, how and what to be engaged in as "work," how to create a family, ethical principles for conduct, and a thousand other things.

> "The meaning-regulative principles of a culture that are passed on to its members may be what makes a culture a culture, what gives it its distinctive stamp." (Kegan, p. 207)

Culture's Meta-State Levels
If a culture is a "logical level" in the mind, one that you set as a meaning-making context, then you construct your social realities by meta-stating them into existence. Given that, as you now detect these cultural meta-states, you are able to work effectively with cultural phenomena. I discovered the relationship between meta-stating and cultural analysis in the work of John Searle in his classical book, *The Construction of Social Reality* (1995). This led to the development of applying the Meta-States Model to cultures, the cultural awareness, and to cultural change.[1]

In that work, he created a model for how to think about, and work with, and how to understand cultures as the frames that govern groups of people. His model also identifies the phenomena that results from the construction of a culture. As a result, we can now use his formula to work methodically in recognizing and constructing higher cultural levels and realities. This model enables us to model the social reality experiences that otherwise we might find quite confusing.[2]

Figure 8:1

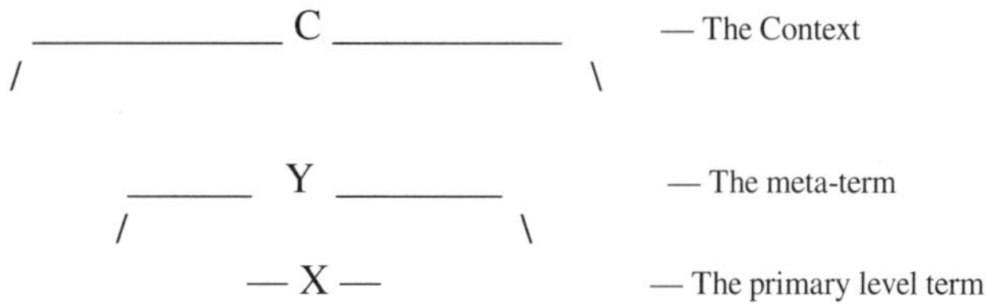

Searle's formula for the structure of a cultural reality is summarized in the following statement: *"X counts as Y in C."*

-     The **X** here is a primary level activity, behavior, or response. Searle uses the terminology "brute fact" to designate some empirical fact that you can see, hear, or feel. X is the primary state (Figure 8:1).
-     The **Y** operates as a meta-term classifying and categorizing the **X** and all of this happens in a given **C** (Context). Y is therefore the meta-state as a frame—an interpretative meaning that classifies the X experience. And C is the next level up meta-state or frame.

Now the **X** fact that belongs to the world, that we can all empirically validate, is just that—a see-hear-feel fact. But what does it mean to the people who have come to endow it with a certain meaning that characterizes from their way of life (e.g., their culture)? Culturally the **X** can be interpreted, categorized, and constructed as a social reality when it is given some **Y** meaning. So it is framed as a **Y** that is, a meta-term. Yet this is not universal. It only occurs within a given context (**C**) as described by those within that community.

Now for some examples.   At the primary level of brute facts *a piece of paper* printed in any given country is recognized and *counts* as money (an X meta-term) when

> Searle's formula for the structure of cultural reality:
> *"X counts as Y in C."*

within that country the government elected or inherited designates certain printing presses as printing the paper that represents in various denominations the money of that country.   So that paper (**X**) in that country (**C**) *counts as* **Y** (money).   It doesn't count as valid "money" elsewhere in other contexts.   Elsewhere it cannot be used for purchasing or exchange, it first has to be converted to the currency of the other country.

Another example from Searle.   From Fido the dog's point of view, a ball being kicked around by men or women running around in a field is just that—a ball being kicked around.   And if the ball goes over a certain white line marked on the field, all of these brute facts are just that —ball, kicking, white marks, etc.   It means nothing more than what it is at the sensory level.

Yet in various human cultures the ball crossing over a line marked on the field (X) could possibly *count as* "a point" or a "goal" (Y) in a football game (C).   It could possibly mean that if all of the context criteria are met.   If a man kicks the ball so it goes over the line during a "practice session," then it is not an official "point."   It doesn't count for anything.   The *context* has to be a game, an official game, a recognized official game, after the official beginning of the game.   Also, if a fan from the bleachers jump over the wall and run out onto the field and kick the ball and it goes over the line, that is *not* a "point."   Nor does it count.   The man was not an official "player" in the game.

The context governs the meta-terms—the meanings we give to the brute facts.   And that context is full of conditions, rules, criteria, prerequisites, understandings, etc. The cultural phenomena that can arise and emerge does so within the contextual boundaries and frames that determine what it means, when, to whom, under what conditions, and so on.

Context and context-of-context, and so on, then enables us to do some very elegant meaning-making as a group or community.   Now we can create cultural meanings at multiple levels and thereby generate a complex set of meanings that make up our social reality. All of this also enables us to create many different facets of meaning in a culture as the content of our cultural life. John Searle lists the following as specialized cultural meanings that we create and assign in a society:

- *Status and roles* to people, situations, events.
- *Functions* of those roles and status standings. These become roles that indicate the structure or landscape of that culture. In a ball game, there are coaches, referees, the ball commission, etc. In the printing of money there are official designations for what holds the status of money, who certifies a printing batch, etc.
- *Status-functions.* We can assign the right, privileges, obligations, and responsibility for certain performances and operations.
- *Speech Acts.* We can designate certain verbalizations as speech acts which creates social reality: "I pronounce you man and wife," "I crown thee the Queen Elizabeth," "I call this meeting to order..." etc.

Cultural Meanings

Now the reason that "culture" hardly seems like an internal frame of mind, a meaning internally constructed, is that we are quick to externalize and embody our "cultural" frames. That's why *culture is a socially shared meaning that is externalized in behaviors and performances.* Yes, it is constructed in "the mind" of a group of people. Yet there is no *mind* of a group separate from all of the individual *minds* of all the people of that group. So where is this *group mind* in which there are social constructions of meaning?

Since the place where cultural meanings exist lies *within the minds of all of the individuals,* what we are actually talking about is *shared meanings.* To share a meaning with another person is the foundational step of creating a cultural meaning. Then it is a matter of multiplication— three people sharing a way thinking, an attribution of meaning, an interpretive pattern. Then 100, 10,000, five million, 3 billion. Then like a gene that replicates itself we have memes—cultural ideas as frames that similarly act in a way that reminds us of self-replication.

Cultural meanings grow, develop, and expand as people share their ideas, generate a common vision, and set an intention that they collaborate to make real. Creating new cultures, cultural frames, cultural expressions, and so on is actually a simple and inevitable process. There's nothing mysterious about it. And when people stop valuing something, when they no longer want to achieve a particular outcome, that culture as the way life has been cultivated begins to decay. It weakens, it begins to dissolve and eventually disappear. This is true of a small family culture, of a business culture, or of a national culture.

Cultures of Meaning

Now when it comes to cultures of meaning, there are thousands of them— there are as many cultures built around some specific meaning as there are meanings among us humans. On the toxic and destructive side, there are cultures of violence, cultures of greed, humiliation, bullying, depression, helplessness, the Hollywood culture, etc. On the constructive and positive side, there is the culture of optimism, sports, Olympic games, higher education, music, art, democracy, etc.

Wherever we humans gather, we are always designing ways of living around experiences and values and thereby creating cultures. We then externalize our understandings, values, beliefs, morals, ethics, into rituals, ceremonies, habits, etc. so that they then become the context or environment in which we live. Eventually we may forget that some person or persons created the meanings and treat the external culture as if a real thing with a life apart from the meanings.

Stories— the Narrating of Culture

Now the most common way that we transmit cultural meaning is through the meaning-making that is inherent in telling stories. A story provides a flesh-and-blood expression of beliefs, values, understandings, morals, ethics, etc. Stories provide a narrative of a set of actions, characters, goals, along with a plot. What story has been told about you, about your family, about your family's history, and so on? Is it a respectful story? A desirable story? Is it a problem-saturated story? A story that you are ashamed of? A story feeding revenge and hatred? Are you ready to re-author for yourself and those around you a more liberating and empowering story? I will return to this subject later in chapter 15 and suggest ways to use story for creating new meanings and cultures.

Neuro-Semantic Learnings for a Neuro-Semanticist

Cultures come and go. They are given birth, grow, develop, mature, grow old, and die as the meanings and significances that they represent live and grow and die. The question then is not whether you are a cultural being. There's no question about

> *Culture is a socially shared meaning that is externalized in behaviors and performances.*

that—you are! Instead the question is this: Are the cultures you live in humane, ennobling, honorable for you and others? Are they fun and loving? Do they bring out your highest and best? Do they allow everybody to actualize their potentials?

- You not only create meanings for yourself individually, you also do so between yourself—relationally and socially. Via meaning-making you create "cultures" as you *cultivate* your mind and heart, and those of your children, and others, and this "culture" exists first and foremost as a "logical level" in your mind. Thereafter you externalize these cultural meanings. You are a cultural meaning-maker! So what culture have you created for yourself up until now? Take a look and identify the cultures you have accepted and/or created.

- You externalize the logical level of meaning about yourself in relationship to others and to groups in writings, architecture, rituals, rules, laws, etc. This makes it easy to forget that culture is an internal thing. Take time this week to begin to see afresh the various cultures that you live inside of and ask quality control questions about them.

End of Chapter Notes:

1. John Searle, *The Construct of Social Realities.*

2. In Neuro-Semantics we have an entire training manual on "Cultural Modeling" using Seale's work as well as that of Korzybski and Bateson.

PART II

THE

PERFORMANCE

OF MEANING

FORECASTING

THE PERFORMING MEANING

CHAPTERS

Now that you have explored Part I which focused on *The Dimensions of Meaning,* it's time to turn to Part II, *The Performance of Meaning.* Now that you know how to recognize meaning in all of its forms, levels, dimensions, and so on, the time has come to ask (and answer) a new series of questions:

- What meanings can I find and/or create that will enrich and enhance my personal life?
- What are the best meanings that I can construct for my driving needs? For my sense of self? For my highest sense of self?
- For what I can devote myself to doing?
- How I can discover what something means to someone?
- How can I detect the meaning that people give to something?
- How can I deframe meaning, frame meaning, and reframe meaning?
- How can I create the most powerful, profound, and useful meanings?

In Neuro-Semantics we do not merely explore meanings at an intellectual or academic activity, we also perform meaning. Why? There's an important reason that we do this. *Namely, meaning must be put into action to become real.* We enact meaning to make it "real" in our lives. When you do this, you come alive to your highest meanings which, in turn, makes your life full-of-meaning (meaningful).

How do you do *enact your meanings* so that you make them neurologically real? You will detect the meanings that you have inherited and absorbed, check them for quality, frame and reframe them so that you choose the best meanings to actualize. You will *apply* the meanings that best enhance life for yourself and others. You will find ways to use your bodily movements, your speech, rituals, storytelling, questions, etc. as ways to apply meaning. Performed intentionally these expressions become enactments of meaning and then your experiences become meaningful —full-of-meaning.

There's a lot of ways to *perform* meaning. Meaning can be performed by asking questions, asking what a word means, what's connected to it, the significance of an event, how it contributes to interpreting an episode, etc. Meaning can be performed by setting up conditions in life, rituals, ways of being in the world, by environment, etc.

Even expressing yourself is an act of meaning construction as you are constituting your Self as a construct according to some meanings that you use as you experience and identify yourself. This makes your self meanings critical as those are the meaning s by which you create and recreate yourself.

Now the most unique thing about meaning is that *it naturally seeks to be actualized within you.* Any and every system of meaning will naturally seek to be expressed in thinking, feeling, speaking, and acting. You, as the rest of us, have an innate self-actualization tendency that drives this.

A central way that you perform meaning is via your conversations. By your conversations you externalize the meanings that you have adopted and created. *What* you talk about and *how* you talk translates your meanings and creates your style of social interactions. The kinds and qualities of conversations that you engage in not only expresses your meanings, *it performs them.* Now you can consider the kind of conversations that you engage in with others in terms of what you are performing via them. So what are you actualizing?

     Conversations of problems, powerlessness, helpless, victimhood.
     Conversations of agency, empowerment, significance.
     Conversations of negativity, pessimism, learned helplessness.
     Conversations of discovery, curiosity, wonder, exploration.
     Conversations of arguments, debate, fight, conflict.
     Conversations of collaboration, allegiance, loyalty, cooperation.
     Conversations of requests, invitations, exchanges.
     Conversations of promises, acknowledgments, commitments.

> Conversations of plans, strategies, outcomes.
> Conversations of optimism, hope, anticipation, inspiration.
> Etc.

To discover this, simply reflect on the conversations that you have and that you live in. This will enable you to determine the meanings that you are currently living. That's because when you talk, you are literally *in-forming* yourself and others—*forming* yourself from the inside out.

Performing or enacting your meaning is inevitable. You cannot *not* do this. Because you are a neuro-semantic being, the semantics of your mind and understandings will inescapably be translated into your neurology. This internal actualizing drive guides your mental-emotional, semantic-somatic system to self-organize.

Given all of this, in the following chapters I our focus will be on how you can actualize your highest and best in the following domains:

Chapter 9:   Your Biological Needs and Vitality

Chapter 10:   Your Self as a Person

Chapter 11:   Your Higher Self

Chapter 12:   Your Reflective Awareness or Mindfulness

Chapter 13:   Your De-Construction of old Meanings

Chapter 14:   Your Creativity in Inventing and Innovating

Chapter 15:   Your Narrative Meanings

Chapter 16:   Your Communication Excellence

Chapter 17:   Your Modeling of Excellence

With this forecasting of what you will experience in the following chapters, you'll learn how to begin to think and act as a Neuro-Semanticist. If you're ready for this, on to the exploration of how to *perform the meanings that you create.*

Chapter 9

ACTUALIZING

YOUR BIOLOGICAL NEEDS

"... man, by having become a human being,
in no way ceases to remain an animal."
Viktor Frankl (1969)

You are an animal! No, I'm not cursing or insulting you, I am simply describing one aspect of your embodied experience. At the biological level of your needs, the driving impulses that you have within your body are animal needs. They are the same needs that animals experience. So, who are you? You are a biological being who's most fundamental drives consist of the homeostatic needs of your neurology. Yet what distinguishes you as a human being is that these drives do *not* operate apart from your concepts, your understandings, your beliefs. For you, the unique factor is that your animal drives are governed by your meanings.

That explains why, in the process of actualizing meaning, the place to begin is with *the meanings* that you give and experience relating to your basic biological needs. Traditionally we have called these biological needs the human "instincts." But they are not. They are not "instincts" at all if by that term we mean that you already *know* what the drive is and how to fulfill it.

Animals have instincts in that way; we humans do not.

That's why Abraham Maslow called these so-called "instincts" by another name. He called them *instinctoids*—they are instinct remnants that drive us, but which lack the content knowledge that characterizes animals. Unlike the animals, we innately do not know what the needs are or how to gratify them. We are not born with that kind of understanding or programming. Unlike the animals, we have to learn what they are, how to satisfy them, and how to develop the actual skill of gratifying them.

If we have an "instinct" it is the instinct to learn, to discover, and to create meaning. That is about the only instinct that we have. The meaning that you give to your somatic experiences (your drives) determines the quality of your well-being in your body and your emotions. This raises numerous questions:

- What is the relationship between meaning and your biology?
- Is there a relationship?
- Does your meaning-making influence your biology?
- Do the meanings that you give to your biological needs have an affect on them?
- If so, to what degree? And how?

Chapter five, *The Embodiment of Meaning,* noted that the meanings that you and I create greatly influence our biology, our so-called "instincts," our health, longevity, etc. When I began my search into Self-Actualization Psychology, I revisited Maslow's work which culminated in his classic *Hierarchy of Needs* (1941, 1954). That's when I realized something critically important about my biological needs and yours—*they are informed by our meanings.*

Yet expressing it in that way actually severely understates the degree and extent that meanings inform and govern biology. So to express this in a more shocking way, in a way that I hope will surprise and awaken you, even shock you, I usually put it like this:
The meaning you give is the instinct that you live.

Now if this statement strikes you as incredible and if you are asking, "What does that mean? How can that be? How far does that go? Then this chapter is for you as I'll answer these questions.[1]

The Biological Needs

In his classical work, *Motivation and Personality* (19564), Maslow identified the large range of "needs" within human nature that drive us. These needs describe the

> *The meaning you give is the instinct that you live.*

levels of biological urges as the instinct-remnants or instinctoids which create the motivation that is natural within people. Maslow separated these into five categories—classes of needs which emerge one after the other as they are sufficiently gratified:

> 1) *Survival:* air, food, water, shelter, sleep, sex, etc.
> 2) *Safety and security:* stability and order.
> 3) *Social:* love and affection, connection and bonding.
> 4) *Self:* importance, respect, dignity, recognition, acceptance.
> 5) *Self-Actualization:* knowledge, meaning, beauty, music, justice, mathematics, equality, contribution, making a difference, etc.

Maslow noted that these needs are hierarchical in that the lower the need, the more it exercises a driving, controlling, and governing influence and that it must be gratified to some extent for the next class of needs to emerge. He also noted that the need does not have to be completely or perfectly gratified. It might only be gratified at 30% or 50% for the next level to begin to emerge in consciousness.

Deficiency is the mechanism that governs the first four levels of the human needs. These foundational driving needs emerge and drive you when you lack what you need—when you are deficient of that which gratifies the need. And, when the need is satisfied, the gratification of the need causes the drive to go away.

Then, after you experience these needs over time and learn how to cope with them— knowing what the *drive* is, what it is calling for, how to meet that need with a "true satisfier," and to do so sufficiently (an adequate amount of the satisfier)—the importance of the need afterwards depend on what you believe about the need. This introduces the realm of meaning as interpretation and understanding. It speaks about how the need can operate *symbolically* for something else. Hence you can interpret your need for food symbolically fulfilling your need for love, affection, dignity, success, etc.

Maslow danced around this awareness without making it fully explicit. And because he did not, he missed the critical role that *meaning* itself plays as the determiner in the whole process. Now true enough, he came very, very close to recognizing it and was right on the verge of recognizing it. But he was only close. So prior to his early death at 62 years of age, he did not explicitly recognize the role of meaning attribution in how we experience the drives or needs. I wrote about this in chapter 7, "Maslow and the Role of Meaning" (*Self-Actualization Psychology* (2009).

"Needs" Without Content Information

Question: What are the human needs that drive you so powerfully? *Answer:* They are the inner biological impulses which urge you to feel, to act, and to respond. They are raw urges that move you but which lack any informational content. So while you feel and act or react, you don't know what the urge is, what it means, or how to gratify it. At least, you do not innately know. You have to learn. At birth these drives are blind motivations in you and you are without an inherent understanding about these motives. You are blind to them until you learn to interpret them in some way.

This explains why you have to kid-proof your house when a baby is born. The baby doesn't *know* what is food, what to eat, what to put in his or her mouth—and so once the baby is able to put things into his or her mouth—anything and everything is fair game! The baby does not know. We have to teach the child what to eat and what not to eat. The same is also true for every other driving need—what to drink, what the discomfort of sleep means, the discomfort of being wet, etc. Humans, unlike animals, do not innately "know" how to meet the biological needs as animals "know" how to meet their needs.

That's why the human adventure involves learning how to accurately and adequately give the driving urges, that you sense and feel, meanings that will serve you well. You have to learn how to give it the basic meanings of identity, cause, and significance:

    1) *Identity meaning:* What is it? How do we describe it?
    2) *Causational meaning:* What does it do? How does it work? What can we use it for?
    3) *Significance meaning:* What is its value or importance?

When you do not know *what a thing or process is*, you won't know how to respond to it. Should you approach or avoid? Is it safe or dangerous? And without knowing what it is, you also don't know how it works. How does it function? What operations can it be used for? What does a person have to know or what skills develop in order to handle it properly? And without knowing its identity or causes, you don't know its significance.

The adventure of meaning begins with these questions and understandings. Then, as you learn to give the meanings that you do to your inner drives and impulses, the meanings that you give endows your inner drives with a motivational direction and focus. Your adopted or created meanings then govern how you express that drive. Your meanings determine how you feel and your intuition about living that drive. First you load your needs with meaning, then you live your drive. *The meaning that you give is the instinct that you live.*

If, on the other hand, you encounter one of your biological needs and are not able to make sense of it, then as with anything that you can't make sense of, you will feel confused, disoriented and will try to adjust yourself by accommodating yourself to things or assimilate it into yourself or defend yourself against it and feel threatened by it. The disequilibrium that then occurs is a problem of meaning. You don't know what it is and so you don't know what to do in response to it. Learning to cope with needs requires that we know what it is first.

As an example, consider what happens if you over-load something as biologically simple as food. The things you put in your mouth and chew and digest can be loaded with so much meaning, that you then begin to eat for those psychological meanings more than the biological nourishment or even, rather than its biological value. If you semantically load food or any particular food (a cookie, ice-cream, etc.) with such meanings as "the good life," "reward," "being a good boy," "success," "de-stressing," "mood food," "the sweetness of life," "being loved and valued," "comfort," "avoidance of feeling inadequate or angry," etc., then you can create a tremendous motivation—one that increases the probability of obesity. Then when a person sees the dis-value of over-eating or eating too much junk food, and tries to stop himself, he will more than likely find the loss too much. *The meaning that you give is the instinct that you live.*

Or consider what happens if you give food the opposite kind of meanings. What if you considered food "dangerous," "a threat to your self-image," "loss of control," "fatness," etc.? then you can probably create a good case of anorexia nervosa or bulima. Then even if the person becomes so thin that it threatens the healthy functioning of various organs or the dissolution of gums, the person still will not and cannot eat. The person's meaning about eating, about food, is so semantically loaded, that their "instinct" goes against biological health and well-being. *The meaning that you give is the instinct that you live.*

In all of this, when you semantically over-load any driving need, you can create biological addictions. This is true of the obvious addictions to drug and alcohol, to gambling, obesity eating, eating disorders, and also of other addictions— shopping addictions, approval addiction, conflict fear, fear of risk (risk aversion). An addiction is a semantically-loaded experience which a person's neurology come to feel as a basic biological need.

Instinct-less as a Meaning-Maker

Because you and I are without instincts, without the program of innate content information like the animals, we are born ignorant. Practically this means that we simply do not how to meet our basic human needs. We have to learn by receiving information from the nurturing community within which we develop. Later we learn by inventing the meanings that we come to believe and that we choose to believe about our needs. That's why the meaning that you give is the instinct that you live implies something quite incredible— *You are the creator of your instincts.* Whatever feels right to you about any innate impulse or need, it feels right, natural, and intuitive because you created a meaning and then you have embodied it. Your intuitions and "instincts" are not given, nor are they infallible. They are the result of the meanings that you have received growing up and the meanings that you have learned in the contexts of your experiences.

So as you create meaning, you endow your soma (your body) with the content information that it will then seek to actualize. Your somatic systems (your neurology, physiology, organs, etc.) are designed to actualize the information. It will take information that is false and inaccurate and do its best to make it real. Of course, this will generate lots of psychosomatic problems and can create all kinds of problems.

The actualizing drive isn't constructed to test or question the incoming information. You have to learn to do that so you learn to think critically. The drive is only designed to seek to actualize the information you accept. The job of testing or questioning the information belongs to our conscious awareness.

Actualizing Your Highest and Best

To actualize your highest and best in regard to your biological needs, you need to answer the three meaning questions about identity, cause, and significance.

> Because the meaning that you give is the instinct that you live—*You are the creator of your instincts.*

1) *What is this need, drive, or impulse?* What is the requirements for well-being that it is seeking? At what level on the hierarchy is this need?

2) *What is this drive seeking to do?* What is it seeking to achieve for you? How is it adequately gratified? What are the true satisfiers for this drive— the satisfiers that will make the drive go away when gratified? What are some of the false satisfiers within your culture that you need to be alert to?

3) *What is the value, significance, and importance of this drive?* What understandings and beliefs about it enable you to give it the right amount of meaning without semantically over-loading it with too much meaning or distorted meanings?

Knowing the answers to these questions enables you to give the need the right amount of meaning, thereby informing you how to effectively cope with the drive when it arises. And coping effectively leads to the drive vanishing from awareness in your consciousness thereby freeing you to focus on your higher needs.

Self-Actualization Assessment Scale

How are you doing with your basic needs? One way to find out is to use the Self-Actualization Assessment Scale that I developed with Tim Goodenough. I have included a diagram of this scale here for you to use for your own self-analysis. What follows after the summary are some of the basic instructions for how to read and fill out the assessment scale.

Neuro-Semantic Learnings for a Neuro-Semanticist

What learnings have you made as you read this chapter that will enable you to more effectively handle the innate impulses that create your sense of energy, vitality, and motivation?

1) If you are the creator of the "instincts" that you feel in your body, if these impulses arise from and result from the meanings you have created and programmed about them from your understandings and

interpretations, then what is the quality of these instinctual drives within you? How are you doing in terms of gratifying them effectively?

2) Given also that the meaning you give is the instinct you live, then how healthy are your instincts? Use the Self-Actualization Assessment Scale to find out. What shifts or changes in your meanings do you need to create to manage your "instincts" better?

Self-Actualization Assessment Scale

Developed by Dr L.Michael Hall &
Tim Goodenough

Meta Needs

Cognitive needs: to know, understand, learn
Contribution needs: to make a difference
Conative needs: to choose your unique way of life
Love needs: to care and extend yourself to others
Truth needs: to know what is true, real, and authentic
Aesthetic needs: to see, enjoy, and create beauty
Expressive needs: to be and express your best self

Self

Importance of your voice and opinion
Honor and Dignity from colleagues
Sense of Respect for Achievements
Sense of Human dignity / Value as Person

Social

Group Acceptance / Connection
Bonding with Partner / Lover
Bonding with Significant People
Love / Affection
Social connection: Friends / companions

Safety

Sense of Control: Personal Power/ efficacy
Sense of Order / Structure
Stability in Life
Career / Job Safety
Physical / Personal Safety

Survival

Money
Sex
Exercise
Vitality
Weight Management
Food
Sleep

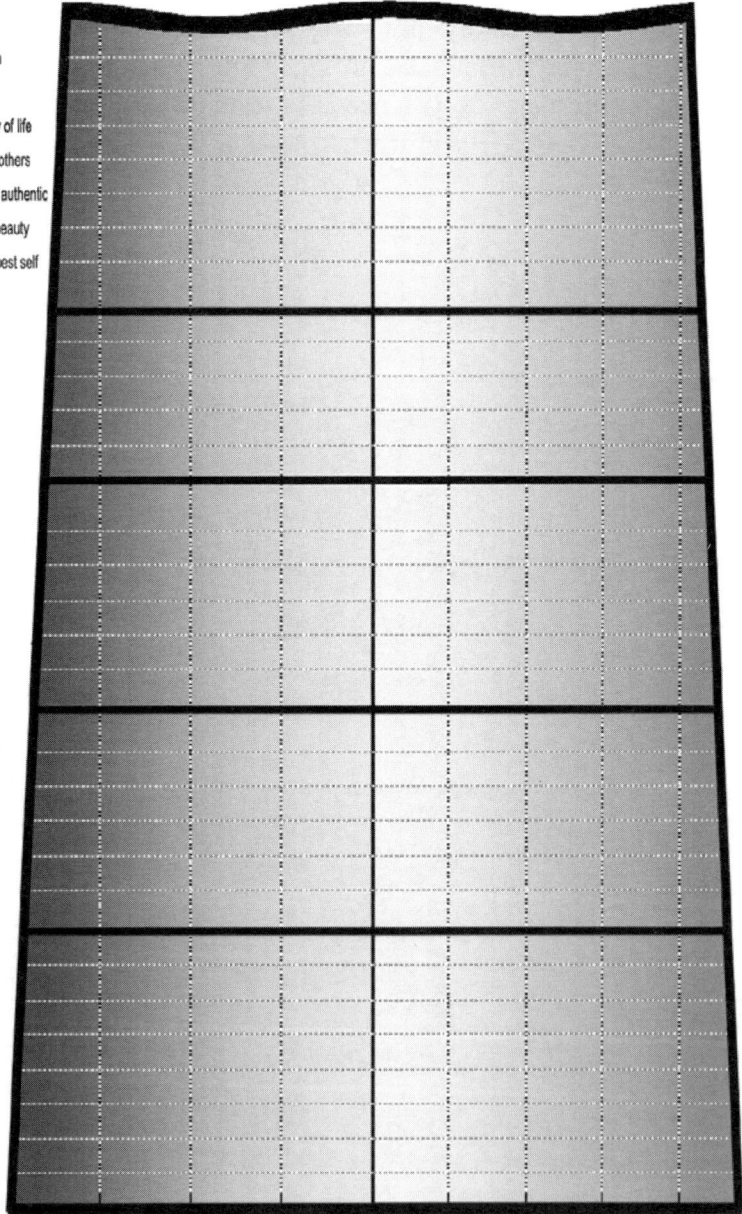

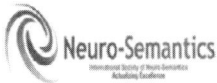

Neuro-Semantics
International Society of Neuro-Semantics
Actualizing Excellence

Dysfunctional	Extremes	Not getting by:	Doing OK	Getting by well	Doing Good	Optimizing	Maximizing
Neurotic	Too much	Cravings	Getting By	Feeling Good	Thriving	Super-Thriving	At ones very best
Psychotic	Too Little	Dissalisfaction	Normal Concerns				

THE SELF-ACTUALIZATION
ASSESSMENT SCALE

How to Use the Assessment Tool

1) Start at the bottom and work up.
Begin with the survival needs and work up the diagram. The diagram of the pyramid is made up of many continua of needs, several in each category (survival, safety, social, and self).

Use the framework of each line as a continuum that measures your *overall, global, or general sense of efficiency in meeting your needs.* How are you doing? What is your overall sense? Are you getting by? Then you are in the middle. If you are *not quite getting by*, there's some stress and strain in getting your needs met effectively, then you are on the left side—in **the Red Zone.** If you are not only getting by but doing pretty good, then you are to the right of the middle, in **the Green Zone.**

2) View the continuum as a measurement of your overall coping with your needs.
The continuum goes from the far left side and gauge several stages in the process of handling your needs: dysfunction, distortion (coping is at extremes of too much, too little), not quiet getting by. The Red Zone is where the *deficiency needs* are crying out that you are just not satisfying/gratifying the needs well. You are either not using "true gratifiers" (Maslow) or the gratification is too much, too little (the "extremes") or completely distorted and creating all kinds of human dysfunction— neurosis and psychosis.

The continuum on the right side of the middle gauges the stages beyond "Getting by:" getting by pretty well, doing very good, optimizing your

Dysfunctional	Extremes	Not Getting By	Getting By	Getting by	Doing Good	Optimizing	Maximizing
Neurotic	Too much	Cravings,	Doing Ok	Well –	Thriving	Super-Thriving	At one's
Psychotic	Too Little	Dissatisfaction	Normal concerns	Feeling Good			Very Best

coping skills (having some expertise in them), to maximizing them (being absolutely masterful in handling them). No one is completely at the right hand of the continuum. "Masters" can move there from time to time. It is the ideal of where you can reach in terms of effectively gratifying your needs. When there, your consciousness, emotions, and energies are completely freed from that driving need so that you have all of that available for moving up the hierarchy and into the human self-actualizing needs at the top.

3) Mark your default point and your range.
Without identifying any particular context, answer it globally or generally for your life. (We will use various contexts later). Put a check (or tick) where you basically are today. Then put brackets [around where you move back and forth— the range of your coping gratifications]. The check is your default point (use one color for this). The brackets is your range (use a different color for this).

4) Sort for quantity and quality.
As you think about gratifying each need —note the amount (number, volume, quantity) of how many gratifications there are for the need. Then note the quality of those gratifications. Indicate Quantity (amount, times, how often, degree, volume, etc.) with a "**V**" (for volume) and for Quality use a "**Q**."

5) At the top identify your highest life themes, visions, and meanings.
Above the "lower needs" (the animal needs, Maslow) are the "higher" or human needs. These self-actualization needs are where you truly live the *human life.* Here you can live for contribution, justice, fairness, music, beauty, mathematics, making a difference in a given area, health, spirituality (as you define it), excellence, honor, loving, etc.

> What do you live for?
> What is the highest meaning and vision of your life? What do you seek to actualize?

Deepening the Analysis
1) *First Analysis:* First use the tool to get a general picture of your coping skills as you gratify the basic human needs that drive you. Here are essential questions to ask after you complete the diagram:

> Where are you overall?
> How are you gratifying your needs? Doing what? How coping?

Do you live in the Red Zone mostly or in the Green Zone mostly?

Is there a particular level of need (survival, safety, social, or self) that you could address that would provide a real unleashing of potentials?

What have you discovered from this first level analysis? What are you aware of?

Are there any strong areas of deficiency?

Are there any strong areas of optimizing or maximizing that gives you a real resource?

Is there any need that you are not gratifying effectively that's serving as an interference to your self-actualization?

Did you leave any of the need continua blank? Why?

The relationship between Volume— Quality in fulfilling your needs:

Notice where you put the V and the Q for each need:

>   Is the Quality always beyond (and higher) than the Volume?
>   Is the Quality always before (and lower) than the Volume?
>   Do the Q and the V shift around depending on the need?
>   Is the Quality and the Volume always or usually together?

2) *Second Analysis:* Next explore your (or another person's) thinking, understanding, believing, deciding, etc. that sets up the standards of evaluation that you or the other person uses:

>   What do you think or believe about X? (Any continuum need)
>   How accurate do you judge your thinking and understanding?
>   What evaluations have you heard from others about need X?
>   What does it mean to you to "get by?" How do you feel about that?
>   How stressful is it when you are not "getting by?"
>   How stressful when you are in the Red Zone?

3) *Third Analysis:* Another analysis can be around the thinking style used to create and evaluate the need and ways of coping with it. Examine the thinking and evaluating by the list of Cognitive Distortions to detect to what extent they play a role in how you think and cope. [See Chapter 6 on the Cognitive Distortions.]

4) *Fourth Analysis:* For this analysis, imagine yourself "in the shoes of someone who knows you very well." Now fill out a second Pyramid Assessment *from that second-position perspective*

>   How does that compare to your first Assessment?

What insights or awareness does this give you?

5) *Fifth analysis:* Another level of analysis that you can use is that of contexts. If you use a specific context: work and career, home, relationship, hobby, sports, leadership, management, etc., then what new or different information emerges?

>   What contexts are important to you? Identify one and fill out the Needs Analysis again using that context.
>   What new awarenesses or insights does this elicit for you?

Exploring Human Needs
After you have filled out the *Pyramid Assessment Tool,* you can use it to explore in more depth your needs or the needs of a client.

1) *Health and Vitality.* Identify the health and vitality of each need: What level of health and level of vitality do you feel with regard to this need?

>   1) How strong is your need or drive for X?   0 to 10, how intense?
>   2) Is the drive or need at a level that you can handle?   How dominating is it?
>   3) How often do you think about your drive/ need? (Hourly, daily, weekly, monthly)
>   4) Are any of the needs especially stressful you? How much stress does it create for you?
>   5) Does the way you gratify the need create a leash? How does it leash you and prevent you from reaching your higher potentials?
>   6) What activates the drive or need in you? How does it get amplified?
>   7) How do you experience it?
>   8) Are your coping skills able to effectively gratify your needs and leave you with energy and vitality for the purpose of your life?

2) *Meanings:* Identify the meanings informing and governing each need:

>   1) What do you think about need X? [X being any of the needs]
>   2) What do you believe about the need and what do you believe about your coping behaviors?
>   3) What is your criteria and standards for making the evaluation about it that you did?
>   4) Do you experience or seek to experience "the meaning of life" through any of the lower needs? If so, which one? (Example, money, status, friends, acceptance, etc.)

5) At what level do you find yourself most frustrated?

6) What need level do you feel stuck at? Which seems to prevent you from going after your dream and unleashing your highest and best?

3) *Semantic over-loading.* Identify if there is any semantic overloading of meaning creating distortions of the need:

1) Is there any need that you have given *too much meaning*? Too much importance? If so, which one?

2) Is there any need that you have given *too little meaning*? If so, which one?

3) Do you have any limiting beliefs about that need? Has anyone suggest that you might?

4) How much of your mental and emotional time do you think about that need?

5) Do you engage in psycho-coping behaviors? (Psycho-eating, psycho-spending, psycho-sexing, psycho-saving, etc.)

6) Are you facing any negative behavior consequences from your eating, exercising, earning, saving, relating, etc.? (example: health problems, relationship, career problems)

7) What happens to your needs under some/moderate stress?

8) What happens to your needs under major stress?

4) *Contexts:* Explore the semantic environment around the need:

1) What are your meanings and beliefs about the context of any given need?

2) In what contexts do you thrive?

3) In which contexts do you just get by and need more effective ways of coping?

4) In which contexts do you struggle to even get by meeting your needs?

5) *Skills:* Explore your skills for gratifying (satisfying) the needs:

1) With any given need, how do you gratify this need? How else?

2) How effective are you in these coping skills?

3) Which skills need improving or changing? Which are excellent?

4) How extensive is your repertoire of skills for gratifying any given need?

5) What are your very best skills in meeting your needs?

6) How often do you use your coping skills to satisfy the drive or need? How often do you forget to use them?

End of the Chapter Notes:

1. See *Self-Actualization Psychology* (2009) and *Unleashed* (2007) for full presentations on this subject.

2. For more about how we humans over-load food in particular and under-load exercise, see the book, *Games Fit and Slim People Play* (2001).

3. The Hall / Goodenough Self-Actualization Scale for Needs Assessment is designed for as a tool for Meta-Coaches, a tool for identifying where a person is strong and skilled in meeting the basic human needs that drive us and where a person may need coaching. The Scale enables you to identify areas that will facilitate the unleashing of potentials.

Chapter 10

ACTUALIZING

YOUR SELF AS A PERSON

OF VALUE AND DIGNITY

"The greatest discovery of my generation is that human beings,
by changing the inner attitudes of their minds,
can change the outer aspects of their lives. ...
It is too bad that more people will not accept this tremendous discovery
and begin living it."
William James

"The man who regards his life as meaningless
is not merely unhappy but hardly fit for life."
Albert Einstein

Once you have started actualizing the innate motivation of your fundamental biological needs, you will be ready to actualize the next level of your needs. These are your driving needs to discover and develop your real self as your highest self which requires that you will need to know yourself, value yourself, and give great meanings to yourself as a person. Then you in yourself will be meaningful.

If you have first created accurate and positive meanings of your biological needs, you have created accurate meanings about the identity, cause, and significance of your basic needs. And how will you know? Success in this will show up in two ways: First in your ability to *cope effectively* with your needs. Second, you will have plenty of *vitality and energy for living* your life. Having done that, something that has been within you all your life will begin to emerge with a rejuvenating force. Now you will be ready to create great meanings about human nature and yourself as a human being and you'll begin to catch a fuller vision of how you can actualize your highest and best meanings as your contribution.

At this point it should be no surprise that if you want to perform and actualize your best sense of self and identity, you will need to discover and/or create some great meanings about yourself and for yourself. I'm not talking about grandiose meanings or unrealistic meanings. I'm talking about meanings that inspire, that call forth your best, and that give you a solid sense of yourself so that, paradoxically, you can get your ego out of the way. This is the paradox of self-actualization— it is not about you! Self-Actualization comes through you for the contributions that you are able to express and give, but it is not about you.

Yourself as a Self
You were not born a self, you become a self. In fact, you are required to invent yourself and to do so again and again throughout the span of your life. That's because the meanings you have received and created construct your sense of yourself— your identity, and your inward experience of being you. And as with every other construction of meaning, the quality of your self depends on the quality of your meanings about your self. What are the most accurate, enhancing, and empowering meanings for yourself as a person in terms of identity, cause, and significance?

You may have read about The Neuro-Semantic Matrix Model.[1] If so, this probably reminds you of *the Self Matrix*— the core content matrix that holds all of your memories, imaginations, understandings, beliefs, frames, etc. about *you*, you as a person, you in terms of your worth and value as a human being, your self-esteem, and so on.

In self-actualization you become the best version of you. You discover and unleash the possibilities within yourself and develop them so that you make real your highest and best potentials. This requires that you identify and develop the passions clamoring inside that you may not even be aware of or that you only hear as a faint inner voice.

> *You were not born a self, you become a self.*

The Many Facets of You as a Self

You do not just have one self, you have a multiplicity of selves. Here is a short list of some of your selves:

• Self-Confidence	Self-Esteem
• Self-Efficacy	Self-Definition
• Self-Presentation	Social Self
• Cultural Self	Career Self
• Ethical Self	Relational Self
• Musical Self	Recreational Self
• Sexual Self	Gender Self
• Religious / Spiritual Self	Body Self

Distinguishing Being and Doing

The most critical difference in this list is the difference between what you *are* as a human being, and what you *do*. This distinction is critical for sanity. To be sane as a human being, distinguish between yourself as *a person* and as *an achiever* (or doer) of accomplishments. These are not the same thing. The first describes you as a human being, the second describes you as a human doing.

Being leads to *doing*. The more fully you are able to *be*, to be fully and completely you, to live and exist within yourself as a fully valuable, lovable, and precious human being— to own and experience your worth, value, and dignity—the more fully you will be able to *do*— to express yourself, to extend yourself to others, to develop your skills, to experiment, to find out what you can do well, to grow. And, the less you are able to be your self, the less you will be able to develop your doing-ness.

To develop a healthy Self matrix separate your person from your behavior, that is, your self-esteem from your self-confidence. Do that and you'll be able to unconditionally feel worthy, valuable, respectable, and loveable. And that will free you so you can experience the world fully as you act to express these qualities in your experiences. With a healthy Self matrix you can celebrate yourself and value yourself without putting your "self" on the line with the activities that you engage in.

The meanings you map about your concepts of your *self* make all the difference in the world. It determines whether you move through the world trying to become a Somebody or whether your life in the world is an expression of your Somebodyness. In the first case, you put your ego or self-esteem "on the line" with things that happen. You identify and personalize almost everything that happens, especially things that are negative and/or unpleasant. Yet when you do that, you make yourself reactive, defensive, and thin-skinned. The problem here is not you as a person. It is the frames that you are using to map your self as inadequate, conditionally valuable, and unworthy.

Everything changes when you map your Self as inherently and innately valuable, worthwhile, lovable, and having dignity, as a member of the human race, as a Somebody, and with nothing to prove, but everything to experience. Do that and you become free to *be* and to *become*. You then free yourself to explore, to enjoy, and to choose to only identify with the things that enable you to become more than you presently are.

If you map things in that way, it allows you to explore your potentials, to be open and responsive, to be caring and loving in relationships, to be non-defensive about mistakes, fallibility, and vulnerability, and to be creative with your skills and passions. When you move your ego so that it is not on the line, then there's nothing to prove. And when you get your ego out of the way, you free up lots of mental-and-emotional energy which you can invest in others, develop your talents, and contribute.

Meaningful to the Core

Of all the meanings that you make, the most crucial meanings that you will ever make are *the meanings you make about yourself.* In fact, the quality of your *self* meanings are among most important meanings for experiencing a quality life and unleashing your highest and best potentials. After all, the self-actualization process involves you succeeding at being *you*— your best self. It means being all that you can be and living in harmony with your gifts and possibilities.

Given that, *what meanings have you given to yourself?* What representations, words, evaluations, etc. have you attributed to yourself as a human being and as a performer? These meanings which relate to your *self* concept are your most basic meta-states. Mapping this accurately gives you a solid core that centers you in a state of unconditional positive regard.

To frame it with erroneous ideas puts your self-esteem "on the line" with everything that happens to create great insecurity. To make your value as a person conditional on anything (looks, beauty, strength, intelligence, money, status, degrees, family, etc.) constructs conditional self-esteem and dooms you to make everything about you.

Figure 10:1

Rejection	*Acceptance*	*Appreciation*	*Esteem*
Dislike	Welcoming — Inviting in	Gentle openness	Highly valuing as important
Judgment	Non-Judgment	Welcome warmly	Significant, worthwhile
Rejection	W/o endorsement	with attraction /love	Welcome with Awe, Honor
	Acknowledge but no		
	condoning or endorsing		
	— Doing —		**— Being /**
			Person —
	Performer / Achieving		
	Apply to your doing self – body, life situation,		Apply to yourself as a
	social self, experiences, etc.		Human Being.

The solution? Meta-state yourself with great meanings—with meanings that induce acceptance, appreciation, and esteem in yourself. When you do, you center and ground yourself.[2] You then frame yourself as having high value and unconditional worth so that your self-esteem is a given and nothing can threaten your sense of respect.

As a human being, *you are not the problem.* So, stop being the problem. Have problems without being the problem. Refuse to build a monument to some problem by identifying yourself with a problem (e.g., "I am an alcoholic, a divorcee, a failure, etc."). Then you can also avoid the neurosis of acting as a sadistic guard imprisoning you to some problem. None of these things will help. You are more than all your frames and meanings; if there's a problem, *the frame is the problem.* So stop embodying the problem.

Meta-Stating Your Self
The three states of acceptance, appreciation, and awe which you can use

> Of all the meanings that you make, the most crucial meanings that you will ever make are *the meanings you make about yourself.*

to create three grounding meta-states (self-acceptance, self-appreciation, and self-esteem), are connected. How? They are all aspects of *liking* and *welcoming*.

To recognize this, think about a continuum of *liking* (things you like), a continuum of *welcoming* (when you accept and bring something into your world). Now on that continuum (Figure 10:1), notice that at one end is rejection and from there, the stronger the experience grows, the more you move to acceptance (acknowledgment fo what is), then appreciation (throwing a party to celebrate something of great value) and then on to awe (the appraisal of ultimate value).

Figure 10:2 relates the quality of your meaning-making to yourself as a person—the value, worth, or lack of such that you attribute to yourself.[3] The fact is, *how you feel about yourself* is a direct result from the meanings that you construct, invent, and hold about yourself. So how do you do with this? Any cognitive distortions that you use that undermine your innate sense of value and worth, of importance, loveability, potentials? Any personalizing, minimizing, filtering out the positive, awfulizing, etc.? Are you meaningful in your self to your core? If not, then it is just a matter of meaning-making. Here's a pattern you can use to ground yourself with an unconditional self-value.

Meaningful to the Core Pattern
The following questions are the key elicitation questions that you can use to initiate this pattern:
*   Do you have enough high quality meanings at your core?
*   What are the meanings you give to you? How do you evaluate yourself?
*   Do you ever criticize and/or judge yourself for what you are rather than a mere judgment for a behavior?
*   Do you distinguish yourself as a person and human being from yourself as a performer?
*   How clearly do you make that distinction?
*   Is your self-identity, fully robust and vigorous?
*   Do you operate from a state of knowing and feeling yourself with *unconditional positive regard*?

Figure 10:2

Meaning Scale about Self

Quality of Meaning		*Feeling of the Meaning* = Emotion
Awesome	10	Fascination, sacrilize yourself
A Somebody		Wonder at mystery of self
Valuable		Ecstasy about being a human being
Loveable		Engaged in some activity
Unique		Willing to fully express self
		Able to give of self
		Self-forgetful (ego out of the way)
Okay		Normal
Normal		
Average		
		Easily threatened
Nothing special		Must prove self; Big Ego
		Bland
		Self-judgment
A Nobody		Sick of self
Worthless		Self-Contempt, Self-Hatred
		Futility, Emptiness
Don't *deserve* to live		Despair
	0	

The Pattern

The design of this pattern is to enable you to meta-state your self with some great states as frames. This will enable you to create a solid sense of yourself.

1) Create some rich and great meanings for self.

> What meanings would enrich your *sense of self* as a human being?
> Make a list of four great inspiring meanings. What are they?
> What meanings would empower your sense of doing, expressing, achieving?

2) Apply to your Core.

> Go inside to you *represent* your inner self.
> As a meaning-maker, *attribute* your great meanings to your core until a sense of awe arises.
> What triggers a sense of *awe* in you?
> What is so big, so wonderful, so marvelous, so incredible that you stand in awe of it, speechless, in utter wonder?
> What evokes you to stand in reverence of your unconditional value?
> Do you do this with a newborn infant? A kitten?
> As you apply awe to your self as an unconditional valuable, precious, magnificent human being, how strong is it?

3) Apply to your Expressions.

> *Acceptance*:
>> What have you simply and positively accepted?
>> Think of something small and simple that you can easily accept without particularly liking or wanting, but you put up with it.
>> What do you not do well?
>
> *Appreciation.*
>> What do you appreciate? Is there anything that you *really* appreciate? What causes you to melt in appreciation?
>> What do you do well?
>> [If you set up a sliding anchor, check if the person likes the movement of "more and more" to go up the arm or down the arm, then set three kinesthetic anchors.]

4) Solidify and integrate.

> Imagine moving through life in the weeks and months to come with this frame of mind...
>
> Do you like this?
>
> Notice how this would transform things for you...
>
> Does every aspect of the higher parts of your mind fully agree with this?
>
> As you register this state, what self-anchor will you establish?
>
> Are you now un-stopable?

Neuro-Semantic Learnings for a Neuro-Semanticist

It is again time to step back and reflect on what you have learned in this chapter and create your own customized action plan for meaning-making — this time about your Self.

> 1) Of all the meanings that are closest to you are the meanings that you make about yourself. Given the content of this chapter, what do you now understand about yourself as a person? How do you interpret your personhood? What meanings do you use in thinking about your worth and value as a person? How will that now influence you and your self-actualizing?

> 2) How well have you distinguished being and doing? For nearly everyone, to do this requires that you go against your culture— the values of your culture and the way most people think in your culture. What will you now need to do to assert your unconditional value and worth as a person?

End of Chapter Notes

1. See *The Matrix Model* (2003) for a full description of the first content matrix, the Self Matrix.

2. This describes the basic structure of the self-acceptance, self-appreciation, and self-awe pattern that is run in the Neuro-Semantic training, APG (Accessing Personal Genius). You can find it in the book, *Secrets of Personal Mastery* (1999) and other Neuro-Semantic literature.

3. Figure 10:1 comes from the *Unleashing Potentials* training manual and part of the Neuro-Semantic process of giving positive meanings to self.

Figure 10:3

Great Self-Esteeming Lines

I'm happy being me.
I honor my life as a sacred gift.
I am a bundle of infinite potentials.
My self-value is a given; you didn't give it to me; you can't take it away.
I'm made in the image and likeness of God.
I'm made of the star-dust of the universe.
I was born human and don't have to join the human race.
My dignity is unconditional as a human being.

Chapter 11

ACTUALIZING

YOUR HIGHER SELF

"Each person is a unique individual.
Hence, psychotherapy should be formulated
to meet the uniqueness of the individual's needs,
rather than tailoring the person to fit the Procrustean bed
of a hypothetical theory of human behavior."
Milton H. Erickson, M.D.

"Speaking of higher as opposed to lower dimensions
does not imply a value judgment.
A 'higher' dimension just means a more inclusive and encompassing dimension."
Viktor Frankl (1969)

You are made for higher things than the mere gratification of your basic needs. There is within you a higher drive, a biological drive that begins to emerge as you grow, but that only later fully emerges when you have developed healthy coping skills regarding your basic needs. These are your meta-needs that describe and define your highest self-actualization needs—what Maslow called the *Being*-values (B-Values).
* Do you know them?

- Where are you in terms of fulfilling them?
- Have you discovered your uniqueness? If so, to what extent?
- What self-actualizing skills have you developed for these highest transcendental needs?
- Do you know how to step up to your next level of self-actualization?
- Are you ready to leave the realm of deficiency and live in the realm of *being*?

The self-actualization needs, while present within you from the beginning, emerge later since they occur at the top of the hierarchical levels of your biological needs. These are the truly

> "Human existence is not authentic unless it is lived in terms of self-transcendence."
> Viktor Frankl (1969)

human needs. To make these potential needs actual requires a maturity in your body, mind, and social skills. That's why we say that they *emerge*. They emerge as you learn how to effectively cope with the basic needs so that those impulses go away.

List of the Higher Needs:
1) The cognitive needs   — to know, understand, learn.
2) The conative needs   — to choose your unique way of life.
3) The truth needs   — to know what is true, real, and authentic.
4) The contribution needs   — to make a difference.
5) The love needs   — to care and extend yourself to others.
6) The aesthetic needs   — to see, enjoy, and create beauty.
7) The expressive needs   — to be and express your best self.
8) The justice needs — to be just, fair, create equality.
9) The wisdom needs   — to be wise, integrated knowledge.
10) The meaning need   — to experience life meaningfully.

From the D- to the B- Realm
These uniquely human needs moves you from the D-realm (*deficiency-realm*) to the B-realm (*being-realm*). In the D-realm your motivation is a function of deficiency or lack so that when you do not have a particular gratification, you are driven by it. And when gratified, the impulse or drive vanishes. In the D-realm, you want. It is all about getting. Not so in the B-realm, there your focus is on giving. It is about *being* who you are and *expressing* yourself as you *give* of yourself and your gifts. This expressiveness of your unique gifts endows life so it becomes truly meaningful in a human way.

If in the B-realm, your focus and direction is on giving rather than getting, what other differences occur here? First is the importance of meaningfulness. Life here is meaningful via the expression of your highest potentials that you are now actualizing. Previously in the D-realm, life is meaningful by the gratification of the foundational needs. Another difference is the abundance of peak experiences. In the B-realm, living focuses on expressing your potentials and with this comes those ecstatic moments of peak experiences.

Living Your Highest Needs — Meaningfulness

An emergent gestalt results from the discovery and development of your higher *being* or *meta*-needs. What emerges is a sense of meaningfulness. You sense that you have found a highly significant and meaningful reason for living, for what to do with your life.

Meaning-fulness—we are all wired to go after and to create a life that we find meaningful. Even in the smallest facets of everyday life, we want things to be meaningful—we even want them to be full of meaning. We do not want experiences that are boring or trivialized. Things that are only somewhat meaningful, that only have a mediocre level of meaning, or that lack meaning altogether do not nourish us. They do not call to us; they do not inspire us. When that happens, we lose energy and motivation. We lose focus and begin flaunting about looking for something that is energizing. Conversely, it is when you find something that is full-of-meaning, or that you learned how to view in terms of meaning, are the things that make life seem worthwhile and sacred.

As humans beings, we are made for meaningfulness and to that end we strive. We obviously will not endure meaninglessness. We're not made to live a life that is futile or meaningless. Yet even the loss of something meaningful to us poses a tremendous threat t us. If we suffer the loss of love, a job, a goal, a purpose, we are at a point of great danger. To lose meaning is to be diminished and if it continues to experience "human diminition." It is the loss of your future, your hope, your courage, your joy, etc. that you sense that your life is being wasted.

All of this takes the "spirit" out of us leaving us dis-spirited, dis-couraged, hopeless, and as Maslow noted, "an experientially empty person" And when this happens, we suffer a higher level of pathology, not the pathology of our

body, but of our mind and spirit— the meta-pathologies. And this will not do. We need meaning and meaningfulness.
- So what is meaningfulness?
- What does it mean when we say that something is *meaningful*?
- How do we find it or create a life full of meaning?

Thinking at Your Highest — *B-Cognition*

To think about yourself, others, life, and the many facets of everyday life in terms of these higher needs creates (and requires) what Maslow called *being*-cognition. When you do, you see the world in peak experiences through the eyes of *Being*-cognition, through what the ancient philosophers defined as the good life (truth, beauty, and goodness): truth, beauty, wholeness, dichotomy-transcendence, aliveness-process, uniqueness, perfection, necessity, completion, justice, order, simplicity, richness, effortlessness, playfulness, and self-sufficiency. (1971:102).

> "These are also the 'highest' values in the sense that they come most often to the best people, in the best moments, under the best conditions. They are the definitions of the higher life, of the good life, of the spiritual life." (1971: 105)

Now as you move to this kind of thinking which is characteristic at the self-actualization level, the B-cognition, how does that influence or even transform life? How does that affect who are you at your highest and best? What are your highest meanings when you are thinking with B-cognition? Which one/s of the higher needs really resonates with you? Which ones inherently excite you and cause your heart to pound?

Living at the Height — Peak Experiences

By definition, a *peak experience* is any experience that you find highly meaningful. In a peak experience, it is not the size of the event that counts as much as the significance that you find in it. A peak experience is a moment of glory and ecstasy because for that moment, you are "in the zone," you are fully aware of one or more *being*-values that is present.

Because it's clumsy and ackward to speak about "experiencing a peak experience" I will here shorten the phrase to one word and speak about the skill of *peaking*. To peak is to reach the height of the human needs and drives, it is to experience peak experiences, it is to live in the B-realm of the B-values. And what is a "peak experience?" In peak experiences, you feel at peak of your powers, using all your capacities at the best and fullest. You as fully functioning. There is no waste, all of your capacities are used efficiently for a highly focused action.

> By definition, a *peak experience* is any experience that you find highly meaningful. In a peak experience, it is not the size of the event that counts as much as the significance that you find in it.

There is a sense of something being effortless even when you are exerting tremendous effort. There is an ease of functioning. Everything "clicks," is "in the groove." A peak experience is a moment of life-affirmation, a moment of joy, a moment of high intensity full of meaning that validates life and makes it worthwhile.

> "Heaven, so to speak, lies waiting for us through life, ready to step into for a time and to enjoy before we have to come back to our ordinary life of striving." (1968, p. 154)

If a peak experience describes the best moments of a human being, the happiest moments of life, for experiences of ecstasy, rapture, bliss, of the greatest joy, the questions before us are these: Can we cultivate these experiences? Can we develop the ability to intentionally and consciously *peak*? Maslow answered this in the affirmative, "Yes we can." So now we ask the quintessentially practical question, How?

Cultivating Peak Experiences
First, practice recalling, learning from, and model the peak experiences that you have already had.

> "I would like you to think of the most wonderful experience or experiences of your life; happiest moments, ecstatic moments, moments of rapture, perhaps from being in love, or listening to music or suddenly 'being hit' by a book or a painting, or some great creative moment. First list these. Then tell how you feel in such acute moments. How you feel differently from the way you feel at other times. How you are at the moment a different person in some ways." (1968, p. 71)

Peak experiences emerge as the wonderful moments of ecstasy—they operate as rewards of the meta-life and they create a tremendous sense of vitality. And because of this, Maslow noted that peak experiences are intrinsic reinforcers" (1971: 297). Given this, practice recalling them. Practice reflecting upon them to savor the goodness of life which they offer.

Second, recognize the moments of ecstasy as they occur.
The problem for most of us is that we don't recognize peak experiences when they do occur. We overlook them. We discount them. We need to turn this around and begin to look for them and value them. And once you do recognize them, then learn how to recover them, how to foster them for the peak experience insights and visions that they contain. Peak experiences can be utilize for more. They are orgasms of the mind and spirit; orgasms of vitality— an ultimate resource.

> "The severely disturbed do not have peak-experiences; only the emotionally healthy do." (1996: 39)

Now a factor of peak experiences is that they typically do not last very long. Why are peak experiences transient and brief? Maslow said that it is because we are just not strong enough to endure more of peak experiences because they are often overwhelming. They may overwhelm you with joy, surprise, amazement, love, sadness, wonder, etc. And so, if emotionally overwhelming, to cultivate peak experiences, you will want to recognize this and set an intention to welcome the strong emotions they evoke. Doing this you will strengthen your ability to be with the peak experiences longer.

> "'Highest' means also weakest, most expendable, least urgent, least conscious, most easily repressed. The basic needs, being prepotent, push to the head of the line." (1971: 295)

Recognize and Accept the Contexts of Peak Experiences
Maslow said that peak experiences are often found in profound aesthetic experiences, creative ecstasies, moments of mature love, perfect sexual experiences, parental love, natural childbirth, etc. He noted experiments in which he was able to foster peak experiences using music, visual stimuli, words, and suggestions. And he said that it makes sense that a person could use dance, athletic activities, child-birth, mathematics, art, etc. to cultivate more peak experiences. With men, he found that peak experiences were in victories, success, achievements; and with women– in being loved (1971:104-105).

> "It looks as if any experience of real excellence, of real perfection, of any moving toward the perfect justice or toward perfect values tends to produce a peak experience." (1971: 169). "The love of the

body, awareness of the body, and a reverence of the body— these are clearly good paths to peak experiences." (1971: 170)

Peak experiences do not have to be great big experiences or special events. In fact, they usually are not. More typically they occur and are triggered in the smaller moments of life, moments of mindfulness when we appreciate the mystery and sacredness of life.

Peak Experience Detection and Utilization Pattern
Pick one peak experience and do the following:
1) *Describe the feel of a peak experience.*
>   Describe how you feel in the acute, intense, peak moment.
>   As you do, step more and more into the state of that experience.
>   Coach your body as you do: how do you breath, look, muscle tension, walk, etc.

2) *Differentiate the peak experience from everyday life.*
>   How do you feel differently from the way you feel at other times?
>   What is the difference that makes the difference between normal states and this one? Identify as many differences as you can. What are you thinking and believing? What are you perceiving?

3) *Identify yourself with the peak experience.*
>   How are you at the moment a different person than how you typically experience yourself?
>   How do you feel about yourself in this peak experience?
>   How do you feel about the world? How does the world look to you?

4) *Anchor the feel and state of a peak experience.*
>   Set an anchor for this state so that you have more access to it.
>   What anchor do you want to set for this state?

Making it Meaningful Pattern
This pattern is designed to identify those areas that are required if you are to unleash the potentials that you envision for yourself. Perhaps there are facets of the experience which you do not experience as meaningful, but as menial and trivial. This pattern will enable you to use your powers to create rich meanings in those areas.

This pattern is *not* designed to be used for something that is loaded with negative meanings. It is for something that has very little or even no meaning. You find it boring. You find it trivial. You find it as a nothing. Pick something that is a 0 on the 0 to 10 scale.

Elicitation questions:
What do you need to make much more meaningful to unleash your highest potentials? What do you need to sacrilize?

The Pattern:
1) Recall your subject for unleashing.
>   What do you want to unleash?
>   What will you be unleashed *from* and what will you be unleashed *to*?

2) Identify the menial steps involved.
>   What seems like a chore? What is a menial or trivial step that you will have to do to get there?
>   Do you now think of these requirements as trivial?
>   What unpleasant task seems like a chore? A burdensome or tedious task? [Not something that is negatively loaded, a 0 on the scale.]

3) Flush out the meanings of the trivial or menial.
>   What does it mean to you?
>   What else does it mean? How does it mean little or nothing to you?

4) Expand the possible meanings.
>   What else could it mean? What positive meaning could you invent for it?
>   [Repeat this 3 to 7 times.]

5) Choose an empowering meaning.
>   How much meaning would you like to give to these steps?
>   What would be the most resourceful meaning that you could give this?
>   Are you willing to attribute this more enhancing, empowering meaning to these menial steps?

6) Try it on and test it out.
>   Decision: Are you ready to make a decision for these new meanings?

Identity: Will they affect your identity? If so, how? What new ways will you think about yourself?

Validation: Is this good? Will you keep it? Will it be valuable to you?

Meaning Enrichment Pattern

If the quality of your life is a function of the quality of your meanings, then to enrich the quality of your life, you have to take ownership of the meanings that you create and attribute to things so that you operate from richer and more robust meanings, meanings that serve you well. Are you ready for this? Are you ready to develop, use, and expand your powers for constructing rich and robust meanings?

> "Being human is being always directed, and pointing, to something or someone other than oneself: to a meaning to fulfill or another human being to encounter, a cause to serve, or a person to love. Only to the extent that someone is living out of this self-transcendence of human existence, is he truly human or does he become his true self." (Viktor Frankl, 1978, p. 35)

The design of this pattern is to develop a resilient, flexible, and creative mind so that you can quickly create rich and robust meanings, to make and remake your world and reality. Here you will be modeling your own innate ability to create meaning. As you do, you will being finding and using a good example and then extending your creative meaning-making. I recommend use this pattern ten times or more. When you complete this pattern, you will be able to take anything and sacrilize it—give it sacred meanings that will enrich any experience so you find it as highly meaningful and special.

Elicitation Questions:

•   How are your current meanings about what you want to unleash in yourself?

•   Is the object of your unleashing meaningful enough for you? Could it be felt and experienced as more meaningful? Would you like to endow it with more meaning?

In this pattern you access two states and set two anchors. First, you access and set an anchor for *meaningfulness*, and when you do, it will be emotional. If not, keep at it until you find a meaningfulness experience that touches you deeply.

Second, you will be accessing and anchoring the sense of *ownership*. This means an awareness of your powers and your ability-to-respond, to be at cause, to be a creator in your own world. When you find that validate it, confirm it. "You *did* that!"

The Pattern:
1) Identify and explore something that you feel is rich-in-meaning (Climb the meaning ladder).

What is fully rich-in-meaning in your life? What have you over-loaded with meaning?
How do you represent that which is meaningful? How vividly?
What do you call it? How do you language it? What kind of words do you use?
How do you evaluate it?
What do you believe about it?
How do you value it?

2) Experience the meanings fully in your body.

How compelling is it for you right now?
How much do you feel that this is rich-in-meaning?
What do you feel about it?
How much do you feel that? And what else?
How passionate are you about that?
    [Anchor the state of *meaningfulness*. Anchor #1]

3) Own your meaning-making powers.

As you step back in your mind for just a moment, notice how *you* have accessed and created so much passion, how fully are you willing to *own* these powers as *your* powers to create meaning? You created this! Right now! Here. *You!*
How much *more* can you *own* these powers?
    [If some troubleshooting is required here — as the following:]
        What are the components that make up these powers? Your thoughts, representations, etc. Are you willing to expand and extend these powers?
        How fully do you use your powers and skills as a meaning creator?
Are you willing to take full ownership and responsibly for having created their state of meaningfulness?
How would you like to anchor this state? [Anchor #2]

How would you like to anchor the state of your power to create rich meanings?

4) Apply: Identify what you want to endow more meaning in.

Are there any menial or trivial steps in this? How meaningful are these? Could this "nothing" be more meaningful to you? Then feel this and wonder what meanings you can and will create to enrich your experience?

What is your current meaning?

For what you want to unleash, *what* would make your life more enhancing and empowering if it had more meaning?

What event, idea, or situation currently does not seem meaningful or significant?

Are you willing to endow it with more meaning?

Link: Feeling the meaning—see and hear yourself doing X. Has it linked the two? What's happening? [Fire the two anchors and create the linkage, the association of meaningfulness and ownership of meaning-making to the new target behaviors.]

Troubleshooting at this step: If you are having any difficulty here, ask the following questions:

- What new meanings are you giving it?
- What else could it mean?
- Which would be the most enhancing for life and empowering for you?
- Which new meanings will you give it?

5) Step in and fully experience the new meanings and future pace.

When you step in fully, how does that feel?

What would life be like with these meanings?

Are you ready to take these meanings on?

Will you set them?

Are they now yours?

How aligned are you with these new meanings? Any objections against them?

How will you solidify and integrate these as you move into your future?

Developing Your Meta-Needs Pattern

The design of this pattern is to identify, detect, and then develop your highest or meta-needs.

1) Identify your self-actualization mission.
> What is your mission? What must you do?
> What inward requirement compels you from within?
> When? Where? With whom?
>> [Describe this briefly to ground it in specific actions and context of when, where, and with whom.]

2) Identify your meta-needs.
> What drives this for you?
> Which meta-needs are you seeking to gratify?
> Why? Why do this? Why is this important to you?

3) Identify the interferences or any lack in frames.
> What interferes with this? What contaminates the drive?
> How does it interfere or contaminate? How do you know that?
> What do you believe about ... the thing that contaminates?
>> [Climb the ladder of meaning.]
> What meaning do you need to suspend or release?
> How strong and robust is your meta-drive and your mission?
> What frames drive this? Does it need to be more robust?

4) Find replacements.
> What will you replace it with?   Construct new robust frames.
> Enrich them.

5) Install and integrate.
> Experience as a state
> Create an action plan
> Mind-to-muscle it.

Expanding Meta-Programs

The Meta-Programs Model of the perceptual lens informs your brain, body, eyes, etc. regarding *both what to notice and pay attention to and what to delete as you attend to things in your world.* This dual function of a meta-program is responsible for your best skills and your blind spots. The positive side of the perceptual lens —they give your neurology and mind a focus. The negative side is that they induce in you blind spots.

- If you move toward values, you delete awareness about what you are simultaneously moving away from.
- If you sort for the details, you at the same time delete the big picture.
- If you pay attention to your options, you will be simultaneously unaware of and blind to the procedures.

The solution to this is not difficult or complex. It is to re-direct your awareness in a given context to what you normally delete, to give value to that information, and to practice looking for it. Do that and you will begin to expand any and every meta-program. The beginning place is to consciously decide to aim to do so. Once you have made the decision and recognize the value in expanding your meta-programs, some disciplined and deliberate practice will enable you to develop the meta-program as a set of choices that you have full access to.

The Pattern for Expanding Meta-Programs

This pattern is designed primarily for you to expand your meta-program lens, especially those which might be a *driver* meta-program. This will give you more flexibility of consciousness and so increase the range of your choices. If in a given context, you find that you are unable to see, feel, or respond in a certain way and your current pattern undermines your effectiveness, this pattern will enable you to change the meta-program *in that context.* Yet in saying that, it is just changing it in a given context, not changing the meta-program, not taking that choice away from you.

1) Awareness: Identify and check the ecology of the current meta-program filter.

> When, where, and how do you use this meta-program which does not serve you well?
>
> How does it undermine your effectiveness in some way?

2) Describe the preferred meta-program filter.

> What meta-level processing would you prefer to run your perceiving and valuing?
>
> *Contexts*: When, where, and how do you want this meta-program to govern your consciousness?

3) *Model the new meta-program.*
[Optional choice if you find that you cannot fully describe the meta-program and can create a map of what it would be like to use in the context that you want to use it.]

>Do you know someone who uses this meta-program?
>
>If so, then explore with that person his or her experience until you can fully step into that position. When you can, then step into 2nd perception so that you can see the world out of that person's meta-program eyes, hearing what he or she hears, self-talking as he or she engages in self-dialogue, and feeling what that person feels.
>
>What's that like?

4) *Give yourself permission for expanding the meta-program in that context.*

>Do you have permission to expand this meta-program?
>
>As you give yourself permission, what are you aware of? How well does it settle?
>
>If there are objections or fears that you sense, what are they?

5) *Experiment with the meta-program to try it out as you extend it.*

>Imaginatively adopt the new meta-program, pretend to use it in sorting, perceiving, attending, etc. Notice how it seems, feels, works, etc. in some contexts where you think it would serve you better. Even if it seems a little "weird" and strange due to your unfamiliarity with looking at the world with that particular perceptual filter, notice what other feelings, beside discomfort, may arise with it.

6) *Run a systems check on the meta-program filter.*

>Go meta to an even higher level and consider what this meta-program will do to you and for you in terms of perception, valuing, believing, behaving, etc.
>
>What kind of a person would it begin to make you?
>
>What effect would it have on various aspects of your life?

7) *Give yourself permission to install it for a period of time.*

>Do you have permission to shift to this meta-program filter?
>
>What happens when you give yourself permission to use it for a time.?
>
>Are there any objections?

Answer by reframing and then future pace.

8) *Set multiple frames for the new extended meta-program.*
>What ideas or beliefs would support this way to filter things?
>What meaning would make this more significant and valuable for you?
>What decision or intention?

9) *Future pace using the meta-program in specific contexts.*
>Practice, in your imagination, using the meta-program and do so until it begins to feel comfortable and familiar.

Neuro-Semantic Learnings for a Neuro-Semanticist
To integrate the learnings you made as you read and reflected on this chapter, here are some questions for your consideration:
>1) To what extent have you found some of the potentials that are clamoring within you and turned those into your pathway to self-actualization? What are your next steps in your self-actualization of the highest meanings in your life?

>2) Take time this week to run the patterns in this chapter. What are your learnings and decisions from doing that?

End of Chapter Notes:
1. Make sure you have a real button.
2. The questions of step 3 are precise and designed intentionally. Ask them with distinctiveness.

Chapter 12

ACTUALIZING

REFLECTIVE MINDFULNESS

For Discovering and Creating Meanings

> "...all knowledge is self-reflexive in the sense
> that the knower always is a constitutive part
> of his or her own process of knowing
> and much of it is negotiated with others..."
> (*Research and Reflexivity*, p. 115)

A basic tenant in Neuro-Semantics is that self-actualization is a function of meaning and performance. As a synergy of these two phenomena, it is meaningful performance and the performance of meaningfulness. So, if the quality of the meaning is quintessential for self-actualizing, then to actualize meaning calls upon you to *become fully mindful of the meanings that you attribute to yourself, your world, and to others.* In fact, we could say that self-actualization involves actualizing your reflective mindfulness. A Neuro-Semanticist is meta-mindful.

This means that when you begin living the self-actualizing life, you actualize the special kind of consciousness that you have as a human being— your *self-reflexive consciousness.* This kind of consciousness allows you to be aware of your awareness. Then, with each level that you transcend, your expanded awareness enables you to be aware of that level. Having explored this in chapter four, *Levels of Meaning*, it is now time to put it to good use.

Challenge Mindfulness

"Are you conscious?" I asked. And from the response, I could tell that I surprised him with that question. Actually I wanted to surprise him. That was my intent.

> "Of course, I'm conscious!" he asserted and his tone went beyond just being matter-of-fact. He was not sarcastic, not quite, and yet he was not far from it.

"Great!" I said, "And are you conscious of being conscious?" Ah, that was a very different question.

> "Conscious of being conscious?" he repeated slowly to himself.
> "Yeah, I think so. ... Yes, definitely!"

"So you are mindful of being conscious and of the kind and quality of conscious that you have right now?" I asked, continuing the exploration.

> "Yes, I'm pretty sure that I know the kind and quality of my consciousness."

"Good. And if we move up the next level and inquire about how mindful you are about your mindfulness?"

> "Well, now I think you have lost me."

"Yes, I have ... for the moment, but soon you'll catch on especially as you reflect on this conversation."

Ah, *reflective mindfulness*— the state that arises from being able to detect your consciousness and to do so level after level and so to develop and operate from a mindfulness that is reflective, aware, and alert. In many disciplines this is the ultimate state— a state of reflection, of expanded awareness, of transcendence from the normal state of consciousness,

Using your Self-Reflexivity
•   Exploring Meaning
•   Detecting meaning filters
•   Asking meta-questions
•   Using meaning detection patterns

of wisdom. Here it is a skill of your self-reflexive mind and as such, it is a skill that you can develop as you use it to explore and to create meaning. To that end, this chapter (and the next one) is about precisely that—how to explore and to create ever higher levels of meaning —meaningfulness.

Doing so will give you an expanded *frame awareness* and that level of mindfulness will then enable you to take charge of your neuro-semantic system. It gives your control over the principles, beliefs, and understandings that your system will be seeking to actualize.

The Adventure of Exploring

How can you discover what something means to someone? Begin with the simplest of questions and one of the most profound questions. Simply ask, *"What does that mean to you?"*

> To actualize meaning calls upon you to *become fully mindful of the meanings that you attribute to yourself, your world, and to others.*

Now when you ask this, notice if the person speaks about something *inside* as a frame-of-mind and category that determines a frame of meaning or if the person speaks about something *outside* as what it would mean in terms of behaviors, feelings, responses, consequences, etc. This is the tricky thing about the meaning question. You never know how a person will respond to it and where a person will go in response. So notice. Listen; really listen. While we might expect that the meaning question will send a person inside to his or her matrix of frames, it does not always do that.

So notice. Sometimes the "meaning" will be external meanings, especially the person's thinking about the consequences that will occur —consequences in actions, feelings, relationships, etc. Sometimes a person essentially answers as if someone asked them, "What is your definition of X?"

At other times, the person will go inside and identify what something means conceptually. Sometimes this will be at ready access, in the person's conscious awareness. If so, the person will answer quickly. Sometimes it is not. If the person doesn't, if the person looks up and seems to be searching, the meaning that the person is attempting to access will more likely be the frame that governs the experience and outside-of-conscious awareness. In that case, give the person sufficient time and space to discover what it means. Hold that space, that moment—perhaps with silence, perhaps by repeating the question.

Detecting the Meaning Filters

Every meaning that you or I receive and/or develop creates a perceptual filter. It creates a lens by which and through which, you look out on the world. Whether that meaning is a belief, an understanding, a decision, an expectation, a value, a memory, and so on, that meaning—operating within your mind-body-emotion system—creates a perceptual filter. You thereafter see the world in terms of that meaning. Your world makes sense to you as it is colored by that filter of meaning.

Reflexivity - The Meta-State Mechanism

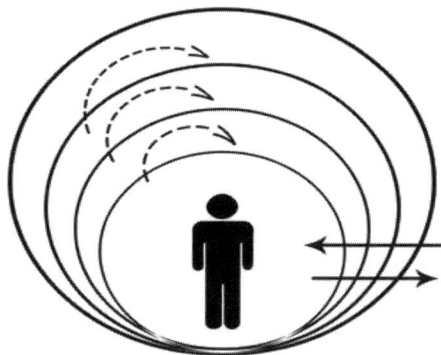

So if you see and perceive things through your meaning filters, how are you ever to detect these meaning filters? This is a kind of catch-22. Your very process of perceiving uses the very thing you want to see! It is like trying to see your eyeball. It is like trying to grab your hand with the same hand.

Well, it may be like that in some ways, yet it is also *not* like that in other ways. That's because unlike your eyeball and hand, with your mind that creates meaning, you have a special kind of mind, you have a self-reflexive consciousness so that you can engage in self-referential activities like detecting and identifying your meaning filters. In meta-thinking, you can learn to think about your thinking, in meta-cognition, you can become aware of the very cognitive processes by which you process information.

How do you use your self-reflexive consciousness in a disciplined way to detect, discover, and expose your filters of meaning? First you set your objective to find your filters. Knowing that you have such filters is the beginning place. And with that you can begin to detect your filters. So plant this question in your mind, "Is this a filter?" "Am I filtering things through this belief? Through this understanding? How am I filtering in somethings and filtering out other things?"

You can also take the list of the NLP Meta-Programs and use them as a filter detector. Take them one by one and as you learn the definitions and distinctions that make up each of those perceptual filters, spend a day or a week really getting acquainted with it— in yourself and in others. This is the process I recommend to Coaches, Consultants, and Trainers who want to have real skill with the Meta-Programs.[1]

Detecting Via Meta-Questions
Now if there is any place where meta-questions are really useful, it is in exploring the meanings and frames in a person's mind. So use the meta-terms for the various facets of an experience to go on the adventure of finding out what something means to yourself or someone else.

There is a particular skill to asking meta-questions—the trick is to be sure to "hold" the context of the previous state for the person. Do this and you will improve the quality of the question and you will simultaneously enable the person to follow your question.

How do you "hold" the context of the previous state? Repeat the words that the person has used and relate your question to that reference as the conceptual context for the question. Let's say you are asking about a particular response that didn't work out for the person, using the person's precise words, *ground* your meta-question with those words to that referent experience.

"So you got that surprising and cutting words from Melissa that you thought were really out-of-character for her, what does that mean to you?"
      "She should not have talked to me that way!"

"Yes, I see, she *should* not have talked to you that way. And that's because it means what to you?"
      "It means she's unthoughtful and inconsiderate and only thinking about herself."

"Okay, so that's what the response that she gave you means to you. The meaning you give it really calls into question her ability to be caring or understanding."
      "That's right!"

"And let's say that's true, so what? ["Let's say that's true" is a phrase that *holds* the concept and invites the person to respond to it.]   What do you believe about that?"

>"Believe? (Pause) . . . I don't know. I just know that she is selfish and only thinking about herself."

"So the meaning you give to her response is that it is an expression of her being selfish and unthoughtful. [Summary offered in a tentative tone of voice so the speaker can correct it, then the summary is posited as true to get the person to respond to that frame.]   Let's say that's true, let's say that she is selfish and doesn't think about you, what do you understand about that? What does that mean to you?"

>"It means that I can't trust her and that being forced to partner with her on this project is not going to work."

"Okay, so you must have a pretty strong belief about people acting in selfish ways.   It sounds like that in your mind it has some pretty severe consequences."

>"Yes, of course."

"And it sounds like, correct me if I'm wrong, that 'selfishness' is a concept that you are highly sensitive to and that really pushes your buttons."

>"Well, yes..."

"And lots of things go into that category, right? That is, you call lots of things 'selfish.'?"

>"Yeah ... maybe too much."

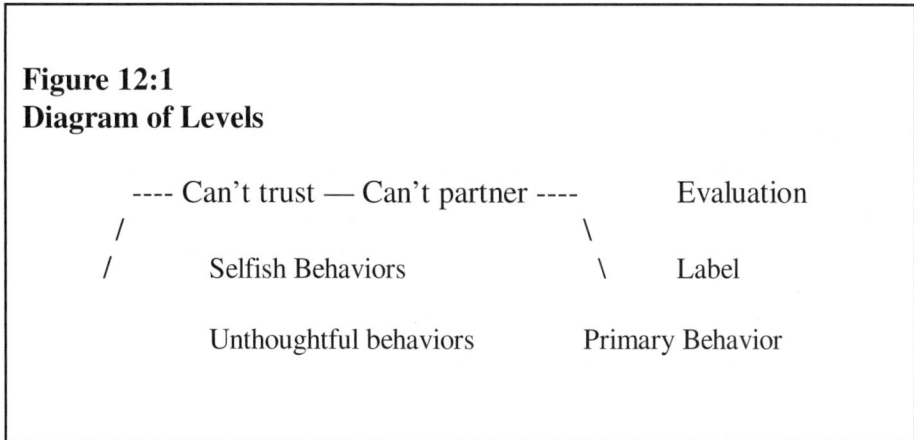

Figure 12:1
Diagram of Levels

```
      ---- Can't trust — Can't partner ----        Evaluation
    /                                   \
   /        Selfish Behaviors            \     Label

           Unthoughtful behaviors      Primary Behavior
```

Holding and Grounding While Questioning

The meta-skill of asking meta-questions is that of holding the referent of your question by repeating where the person is and making sure it is grounded in some real-life external context. Then, holding and grounding, each higher level, you are then able to invite the person to rise above, transcend, or "go meta" to that context, and *including* that context now in a higher frame, to ask a wide-range of meta-questions to thoroughly explore the person's matrix of frames.

Several things results from this process. First, you are providing a context wherein a person can *step back* from his or her own thinking and feeling and gain a larger perspective on oneself. This facilitates a higher level *mindfulness* giving the person a chance to slow down his or her reactions and discover or recognize the frames that are governing such responses. And in doing this, the person moves to a position of being at choice point wherein he or she can make more informed choices about how to respond—choices that fits with the person's highest values and visions.

The Linguistics of Meaning

Meaning is coded in language. While you can construct meaning in the simplest way through the senses—visual, auditory, kinesthetic, olfactory and gustatory representations for coding meaning, most meaning is coded linguistically. So we use language to detect meaning. Use the distinctions and features of language to notice the words, sentences, and linguistic patterns used to construct a linkage between an event out in the world and words that classify, categorize, and define.

Patterns for Facilitating Meaning Discovery

While there are actually many patterns in Neuro-Semantics for discovering meaning, I have chosen to include the following three as those that are among the most powerful. As you learn these patterns and practice using them, you'll be able to get to the heart of things with yourself and others. Practice also will develop your self-reflexive consciousness in its own right.
*   Into the Construct Pattern
*   Coaching for Matrix Detection Pattern
*   Opening up a Belief System Pattern

Into the Construct Pattern

The design of this pattern is to enter a construct system of meaning that you live within to become conscious of it. As a way to let the unleashing to begin, start by detecting the meanings that are now holding you in place and preventing you from moving forward. Here you will enter the Matrix of meanings, explore what's there and begin to use your powers of creating meaning.

The elicitation questions that will initiate this pattern are these:

> What do you want to unleash within yourself?
> What's clamoring to be unlocked?
> What do you want to be unleashed from and unleashed to?

The Pattern:

1) Identify the context for unleashing.

> What do you want to be unleashed *from* and unleashed *to*?
> Tell me about that— When, where, with whom? [Grounding questions]
> What does this mean to you?
> What do you believe about this?

2) Explore the matrix of meanings.

> Climb the meaning ladder on both the attraction and aversion of toward and away from.
> [Map out in the conversation the meanings, and Meaning Matrix of the person, of what you want to be unleashed from and what you want to be unleashed to. The skill you need here is to *hold the level* you are working with. Hold it for the person so he or she can respond to it. Notice if the person answers the question and goes up or tries to escape the frame by escaping to emotions or actions. It's not about the content, it's about the structure, form, or order. Just follow the questions.]

3) Quality control the meanings.

Invite the person to step back and explore of the quality of the potential to be unleashed. This is where you get leverage within the person to facilitate the change.

> What are you aware of? What do you think?
> Does this enhance your life? Does it empower you as a person?
> Are there any meanings that are in the way? What do you think?
> How's your Construct? Is it robust enough to support and drive your unleashing?

4) Decide on preferred meanings.

> What meanings do you prefer?
> What meanings would enhance and empower you in this the most?
> Do you have inspiring meanings about this?
> Do you have a big enough meaning?

5) Confirm and solidify as you future pace.

> So you'd like to have this meaning as your frame of mind?
> Does it empower you as a person?
> Does it enhance your life and enable you to self-actualize?
> Do you like it? How much?
> Will you keep this meaning as your frame of mind?
> How will you remember it? How will you keep it?

A Coaching for Matrix Detection Pattern

The design of this pattern is to enter into someone's Matrix of Frames to find out what something means to them and to move up through all of the Matrix of frames that inform and govern the experience. The intent is to open up awareness for the person about what's going on and invite the person to choice point about what to do. This also is the most basic pattern that we use in the Meta-Coaching process.

The Pattern

1) Identify a trigger in the outside world.

> What are you responding to? What is the trigger? The stimulus?

2) Identify the state you experience.

> What state do you access and experience in the face of that trigger?
> What else is within that state? What else would you call it?
> How much are you experiencing that state?

3) Identify the frame driving the experience.

> What do you think about that trigger? What are your immediate and
> automatic thoughts?
> What does it mean to you? What do you believe about it?
> What does it remind you of? What do you call it?

4) Explore the person's full layers of frames.

> Let's say that's true, so what? What does that mean? What do you
> believe about that?

[Holding each frame, ask meta-questions about it until you get to the top.]

5) *Quality control the matrix of frames.*

Let's set this whole set of frames aside ... and as you step back now and look at those belief frames, meaning frames, understanding frames, decision frames, identity frames, etc., do they serve you well? Do you like them? Do they empower you as a person? Do they enhance your life? Do they enable you to be your highest and best self?

[Save whatever value there may be; integrate those and keep repeating the quality control questions until you get a strong and decisive "no."]

6) *Transition out of that old matrix.*

If you were no longer there and no longer had to think and feel and believe that way, what would you like to think, believe, understand, etc.?

If a miracle happened tonight and you no longer had that response to the trigger, what would be different? And how would you know?

7) *Identify the new state.*

What state would you be in if you were out of that old matrix and in a new place?

What do you call this new state? How resourceful is this new state?
  [Apply until it is strong and robust.]

8) *Identify the new matrix.*

What do you believe that enables you now to experience this new state?

What would be the most powerfully positive belief that would support this? What else?

[Move up the levels creating new frames of meaning about the trigger.]

9) *Quality control and future pace.*

So what would it be like to take this into your future? How much do you like this?

When you have this even more fully in the days and weeks to come, what will that be like for you? Are you okay with this? Any objections? Will you keep this? How?

Opening Up a Belief System Pattern

The design of this pattern is to open up all of the beliefs that hold a single belief statement in place. While beliefs are powerful as "commands to the nervous system," they do not exist alone and often their "power" lie at levels hidden above the obvious belief statement. They operate in conjunction with other beliefs and so operate as a system—hence we describe them as *belief systems*. Where you have a belief, you also have a belief about that belief. And then something about that belief. This pattern is designed to *open up* the belief system itself to find out what are the higher belief frames that support and hold the first belief in place.

The distinction that you will note and use in this pattern is the distinction of the levels of beliefs. Here you are looking to identify the meta-level structure of supporting beliefs that hold a particular belief in place. Here you will want to be sure to hold the first belief in place and then begin opening up the higher beliefs.

1) State Matrix: Identify an action or behavior you want to do.

What sensory-based action do you need to take to make your life much more effective and successful?

Menu list: Exercise regularly, read and study daily, make calls to promote your business, express yourself in a kinder and gentler way, speak up with more confidence, etc.

2) Design the qualities of this behavior.

What qualities and properties do you want in this behavior?

What kind of feeling do you want to texture this action with?

Menu List: Assertive, gentle, caring, thoughtful, sensory awareness, passion, compassion, intensity, relaxation, elegant, professional, etc.

3) Designate corresponding states for these qualities.

What *states* do these qualities imply?

What mental and emotional states would you need to experience these qualities?

Example: If you want passion and excitement then you need a state that corresponds to those qualities. In this case, passion, enthusiasm, ferociousness, etc.

List all of the presupposed and implied states that texture the action in the way that you want it textured.

What would you have to remember or imagine to have that state?

What would you have to represent and how would you represent it?

4) *Meaning Matrix: Identify supporting beliefs.*

What would you have to believe in order to experience that state?
(Access) [Since supporting beliefs need to be strong and robust, make sure you have robust ones.]
Do you believe that? [Confirmation.]
You really do believe that then? [Strengthening the confirmation.]
And what else do you have to believe in order to experience that state?
And as you stay with that belief for a moment, just enjoying it, *what opens up for you* in terms of even higher and more supportive beliefs?

5) *Elicit each belief in order until it elicits the next highest belief.*

What belief supports *this belief?* [To elicit the next higher belief.]
And as you stay with that belief, **what belief opens up** *for you that supports that belief?*
*"And when you believe that, **how fully do you** feel this belief?*

[Keep repeating these questions until the person discovers the higher beliefs that open up in support of previous beliefs. Make sure the person represents vividly enough to *feel* it. Test that by asking the second question. Continue to move up the levels by repeating these questions. In this way you will have the person move up and moving down the levels of his or her mind, connecting, linking, anchoring, using both feedback and feed forward mechanisms. Continue upward through the holoarchy of the person's belief frames. Sketch out the embedded structure.]

6) *Sequence through the entire program quickly.*

Once elicited and designed, run the program of the embedded structure for the entire belief sequence by asking the series of questions:
1) "What actions do you want to perform with more power, grace, elegance" (whatever qualities the person mentioned in step 2)?
2) "And, **what belief supports** that?"
3) "And when you believe that, how fully do you feel this belief?"

These questions that you have iterated over and over should now set off the entire embedded holoarchy, the embedded system of your matrix of belief frames.

> **Holons — Holoarchy**
> A holon involves parts and wholes. A part is a whole in itself and also a part of a larger whole and so makes up a holoarchy in contrast to a hierarchy. As a structure of holons, it is a holoarchy.

7) Quality control the whole system and future pace.

Does any part of you object to having this as your way of moving through the world? (No)

Do you like this? (Yes)

Does it empower you as a person and enhance your life? (Yes)

As you imagine moving through the world with this in the days and weeks to come, can you affirm this as what you definitely want? (Yes)

8) Apply throughout your matrix.

Holding all of this in mind— what state does it induce?

How does it affect your Self, Others, Resources, Time, World?

Neuro-Semantic Learnings for a Neuro-Semanticist

The good news is this: *The meanings that have been governing your life can be discovered, enhanced, and (if you so choose) transformed.* And you can discover the hidden frames that have been driving your experiences and emotions. There are processes that you can use to detect the hidden meanings that are governing and informing the things you feel and the responses that you make.

*   This week, use one or more of the patterns here to expand your meta-awareness about some of your frames.

*   In terms of effective communication, learning how to detect and discover the meanings that another person is attempting to communicate is essential for understanding. So who will you seek to more fully understand this week?

End of Chapter Notes:

1. For the encyclopedia of meta-programs, see *Figuring Out People* (2007).

Chapter 13

ACTUALIZING

DE-CONSTRUCTION

FOR MORE MEANINGFUL OPPORTUNITIES

Once you detect meaning, what then? W*hat do you do after you detect the construction of some meaning that is limiting or inadequate?* Often you can immediately begin adding rich and robust meanings to whatever experience or event you are considering and go directly to actualizing those meanings in your everyday life (chapter 14). But not always.

Sometimes before you can add rich meanings to an experience, you first have to *de-construct (or de-frame) meanings* that are currently activating your neuro-semantic system thereby creating interference or sabotage to your highest and best. The cue for an interference or sabotage will be the sense that something is blocking you, in the way, or that you can't succeed, you don't deserve to succeed, or a sense that there's something dangerous or threatening to move ahead. It will be the sense that there are objections inside yourself that are preventing or forbidding you to go forward.

Sometimes, then, before you can change or add meanings, you have to *undo* some of the meanings that you have created (or accepted), and have been living by. You have to de-construct the old constructions of meanings and release them. The reason for this is simple. There is some current meaning that is in the way that prevents the new meanings or the change of meanings. So this brings us another activity that you'll want to actualize so that it becomes a core competency in your meaning-making skills: *deframing.* This refers to de-constructing the constructions that have been made. And there are numerous ways that you can do this.

Destruction frequently precedes construction. We often see this in urban cities as buildings are blown up to clear the space for a new modern building. We see this in forest fires as nature clears the old growth making way for new growth. So also psychologically, sometimes deframing is required before you can begin creating new empowering meanings.

The Art of Deframing

Just as there is an art of framing as you construct the meanings, understandings, and beliefs that make up a model or paradigm of the world, so there is an art to deframing. And it is equally as important. So, how do you deframe? What are the processes for deframing and what comprises the process of doing this artfully in communication?

1) Relabel.

An easy, quick, and sometimes amazingly surprising way to deframe is to simply re-assign an event, a word, or an experience to a new category. That is, call it something else. And if the new term or phrase captures the essence better or offers more resources for coping with the referent event, then it can undo the original label and re-frame it.

> She is not stubborn — she is tenacious.
> He is not confused—his rich mind is holding multiple perspectives.
> She is not lazy — she is exquisite at relaxing.
> He is not rude — he is unafraid of social rejection.
> She is not bossy — she is decisive and a heroic leader.
> He is not fearful and timid — he is highly aware of the dangers.
> She is not thoughtless — she is selective in her focus.
> He is not a control freak — he values doing it right the first time.
> She is not soft —her compassion sometimes over-rides being tough.
> He is not disrespectful — he has a vigorous sense of humor.

2) *Fragment it with Questions.*

Another way to deframe is to pull the old meanings apart bit by bit so that the gestalt that results cannot be sustained. The best way to do this is to use the exploration questions of the Meta-Model which enables you to create precision out of vagueness. The questioning enables you to loosen frames so that they can no longer glue the older meanings together. By delving into a construct of meaning and exploring it with very curious questions, you can cause a construct to loose its coherency. Then it begins to fragment.

Think of the meaning as a piece of thread that sows together a tapestry of meaning. Identify the thread of the logic that creates a certain meaning and once you find it, explore that thread-of-logic thoroughly. Finding that thread also means that you can begin to pull on it and see if it unravels. It may be that there are knots somewhere which you may have to untie before you can give it a tug which sometimes just a single pull on the thread will cause it to unravel completely the psycho-logic that created it.

Or think of meaning as the foundational stones of your construct. Identify the building blocks that make up the construction that you or another lives within. What are the blocks or stones that make up this fortress or palace? When you find one of the building blocks, ask lots of questions about it so that you loosen it and can pull it out. Which block, when loosened and removed would cause the whole wall to crumble?

The key to deframing by fragmenting with questions is to ask lots of curious questions from a know-nothing state. By simply seeking to understand it and by asking questions about all of its ins and outs, not only do you come to understand the person's construct, but so do they, and if there are places where the construct is weak, that becomes obvious.

You can de-construct meanings not only with primary questions of the Meta-Model of Language, but also via the meta-stating questions that come from the Meta-States Model. When you do this, you are meta-stating a meaning with the questioning state.

This is one of the out-framing processes (#4). Here you simply ask lots of questions, lots of primary and meta-questions as an exploration process to thoroughly understand how an experience works. Do that, and there is little likelihood that the experience will cohere. If it is a diminishing or limiting meaning, the questions will pull the experience apart.

If you and I construct meaning frames by our words, thoughts, feelings, by our references, etc. in the first place, then we can *de-construct frames* by reversing the process. This is the power of asking *the indexing questions* of the Meta-Model. How do you do this?

Ask lots of questions about how the frame and its parts work, how you constructed it, index the when, where, how, standards, etc. This will have a *de-stabilizing* effect upon ill-formed and undesired frames. Enter fully into the person's "text" or frame and explore how the frames and frames-within-frames work. Get as many details as possible as you stay within the other's "logic." As you do this to fragment systemic processes you will be reducing the structure via the reductionist power of analysis.

3) Stretch a frame, even misunderstand the frame.
Frames are just conceptual understandings about things. So as you ask questions, explore how far you can take the idea, how far it will stretch. Find out where it will not stretch, where it does not work.

If a person's understandings about something is too rigid, too solid, then ask questions, lots of questions, then more questions. Do this to provide an invitation so the person begins to *misunderstand* what they thought they understood so well. This will make what was stable, unstable. It will move them from their secure and ordered world to a more chaotic state of mind. Use "What if..." questions and scenarios.

> "Perhaps the best that therapists can do is creatively misunderstand what client's say so that the more useful, more beneficial meanings of their words are the ones chosen." (Steve de Shazer, p. 69)

In the art of inviting misunderstanding, identify and use exceptions, flukes, deviations, and undecidables. This will help to create some slippage between the words and the concepts that make the meaning currently stable.
- Are there any trivial solutions that you have dismissed?
- Is there anything ambiguous about this?
- What is ambiguous about this situation?
- Where is the border of this experience? When, where, with whom, how do you know?

4) Outframe.
When you move above a frame (or step back from a frame) so that you can then think about it, reflect on it, or even bring another idea to that frame,

you are *out-framing*. This is the basic meta-stating process of bringing one level of thoughts-emotions to another level. And when you outframe, you can often bring a higher frame that, in effect, blows the previous frame to smithereens.

In this way you can challenge the old meanings from a higher level—perhaps the higher level of your values or your visions and so run a quality control on the meanings.

If you quality control the meaning with the ecology questions (see chapter 6) you can often torpedo the old meaning in such a way that it is suddenly seen as irrelevant, limiting, diminishing, stupid, toxic, or useless. If the answer to the question, "Does it serve you well?" is "No, of course not!" Then that answer of "no" will work as a rejection of the old meaning. And with that you have probably facilitated a pretty significant deconstruction. There are other beliefs and understanding that can have this same deframing effect, and I'll point them out as we go through the other reframing and outframing patterns.

5) Dis-Confirm.
Suppose you utter a strong and definitive "no" and reject an old meaning or belief that you know is not true or that does not serve you? If you did that, what would happen? Well, from what was just said, you may now realize that you can even more directly simply refuse or reject the old belief. Say "No!" to it in such a way that you refuse it. This is the significance and value of the "Meta-No and Meta-Yes Pattern.[1] The states of *yes and no* are powerful primary states that enable you to cut-off unuseful alternatives from very useful ones, that is literally to make *a de-cision*.

6) Stubbornly Refuse a Frame.
Another deframing process involves using the power of your stubbornness. You do get stubborn, right? And you do know how to effectively use your stubbornness, right? Do you ever make up your mind and won't change it? Do you ever dig in your heels and stubbornly refuse to go along with something? Great! What power you have in this state of stubbornness!

Now let's use it creatively and to your highest values. Access your stubbornness, amplify it so that it is at a peak of intensity, and then for the belief meaning that you know is in your way and does not bring out your best, feel that stubbornness so fully that you adopt the eyes, voice, posture, etc. of stubbornness. Do this until you stubbornly refuse to tolerate the limiting belief or meaning no longer.

When you do this with your stubborn state and then stubbornly refuse a meaning, understanding, or belief you are setting boundaries. You are identifying what is inside and what is outside the boundary. If you have difficulty with this, check to see if you have permission to be stubborn. That experience and state might have been taken away from you and made taboo by parents or teachers.

7) *Release.*

Another way to deframe is to simply release an meaning and let it go. After all, ideas and mental constructs along with tangible things can be released. Everyday you release things: you breathe in and then you breathe out—you release the oxygen. You let it go. You tighten muscles, and then you release the tightening. You eat and drink and then later your digestive system releases the by-products. You open doors and you close them as you say goodbye to someone and let them go.

So, grab one of these feelings so that you know what it feels like to release and be with that feeling. Experience that feeling state until you have a strong sense of it, then "anchor" it with a word, image, or sound. This will allow you to access this state whenever you really need it.[2] Feel it fully so that you can bring that releasing feeling to an old meaning. Bring it and then *let the meaning go.* Say goodbye to it. Breathe it out.

8) *Suspend.*

Then there is the ability to suspend a belief or construct as a way to deframe. You can simply suspend a meaning by a shrug of your shoulder. Do you know that? Is it possible to simply suspend a meaning or is there some way to neuralize what something has meant to myself or someone else? Here is what Abraham Maslow wrote:

> "If you know who you are, where you are going, and what you want, then it is not hard to deal with inane bureaucratic details, trivialities, and constraints. You can simply *disarm* them and make them *disappear* by a simple *shrug* of your shoulders. I know that I am apt to become impatient with young people today who attribute so much power to social pressures and forces. I point out that all we need to do is *pay* those influences *no attention* and then they vanish. ..." (Abraham Maslow, *Future Visions*, Unpublished Papers)

If you have ever "shrugged something off" and treated something as irrelevant than you have the ability to do this with a meaning that has become irrelevant to you.

9) Neutralize.
Frames can be neutralized. It is possible to take a meaning-frame and work with it in such a way that it takes any "emotional charge" out of it. This was the incredible discovery made very early in NLP when Richard Bandler came up with the "Phobia Cure." This pattern goes by several names, the Visual-Kinesthetic Dissociation Pattern. I re-titled it *The Movie Rewind Pattern* several years ago because that is what you do in the pattern—you take the movie that plays in your mind and you rewind it.[3]

10) Reduce.
Sometimes in de-constructing, you do not need to completely eliminate or destroy an old frame or meaning, just reduce it enough so that it becomes less real and less compelling to you. This is where the shifting of the cinematic features of a representation using sub-modality distinctions offers a powerful way to deframe. Take the image, sound, or sensation and simply play with turning its quantity up and down. Turn up the brightness of a picture, then turn it down making it dimmer and dimmer, darker and darker. At what point do you experience sufficient reduction of that image so that you can replace it?

With the sound, turn the volume up and then down, or put it further and further away until the voice or sound is sufficiently reduced. Or turn it all the way down so that it is silenced. You can do this with any cinematic feature by which you code an awareness. You can do this linguistically by using softer type of words. Turn "anger" down to frustrated, then upset, then annoyed, then peeved, then out-of-sorts, etc.

Meta-Model Questioning for Defaming
The design of the following pattern is to use the questions of the Meta-Model of Language on a construct of meaning and to do so until it falls apart.[4]

The Pattern:
1) Identify a frame that you want to pull apart.

Examples include a meaning statement as the following: "I am a failure." "To be rejected or to receive criticism is terrible." "Things ought to be easy." "It's a dog-eat-dog world out there."

2) Frame exploration: Explore the frame by asking lots of indexing questions.

Use the precision language model to question and explore the poor structure of the linguistic statement (meta-modeling). Fragment the statement into the tiniest components.

> What is happening?
> How do you think, feel, and/or perceive that?
> Is it a problem for you?
> How is it a problem?
> How is that problem a problem for you?
> What specifically do you mean?
> How do you know to call it, classify it that?
> When?
> Where?
> Says who?
> According to what standard?
> In what way?

3) Play with the frame by exaggerating it, applying it to the speaker, to others, etc.

We call this conversational reframing or (mind-lining).[5] See how durable, lasting, and solid the frame is by playing around with it. Rough it up, play hard with it. How durable is it when you put it to the test?

Releasing Semantic Reactivity Pattern

The design of the following pattern is to enable you to release yourself from being semantically reactive. How do you do this? You will enable yourself to suspend meaning where you have *over-loaded too much meaning* to your own detriment. The skill you will develop here is that of suspending, neutralizing, and releasing old meanings.

An elicitation question that you can use to launch this pattern includes the following:

Is there anything that you've given too much meaning to, that you have loaded with too much meaning so that it now interferes with your unleashing? What?

The Pattern:
1) Identify something that triggers you to feel semantically reactive.
What pushes your buttons?
What rattles you and gets you into an upset state?[1]
What creates an interference or sabotage to your unleashing? How does it do that?

2) Identify the Meaning Structure.
What does it mean? What does else it mean?
What do you believe about this?
[Use a series of meta-questions to explore the meaning and do so up the levels to expose the semantic structure that holds the semantic reaction.]

3) Neutralize the Meanings.
Do you know that the old meanings are *just* meanings?
How well do you know this?
Now knowing that, what do you realize?
[Neutralize through witnessing, decision to refuse, reframing, making irrelevant, rewinding old movie, or releasing it.]

4) Expand the Meanings.
What else could it mean?
What do others think it means?
What meanings does the most highly resourceful person you know give to it?

Movie Rewind Pattern
When you construct meaning, you put ideas together in a certain order. That order is the syntax that enables the ideas to make sense. Something makes sense due to the structure or order. Conversely, if you change the order or fool around with the syntax, you often miss up the meaning so that it no longer makes sense. This, in part, is what happens within this pattern. In addition to setting lots of frames about an old experience that meta-states it with a new texture, the Movie Rewind Pattern also changes the syntax of the old meanings and thereby messes it up.

Order certain a in together ideas put you, meaning construct you when. Does that sentence make sense? No. Of course not! The order of the words have been changed. But notice the sense that you create in your mind when you read this sentence: When you construct meaning, you put ideas together in a certain order. It's the same sentence. In the one that leads this paragraph, the order of the words are reversed.

The Movie Rewind pattern is designed to take the emotional charge out of how a person' thinks about or remembers an experience. If a mere thought triggers a semantic reaction (a phobia, a panic, or an exaggerated emotional outburst), this pattern enables you to reduce the emotional charge so that you can think calmly about it.

The Pattern
Step 1: Preparation for the pattern.
Are you ready to neutralize an old movie that you have played in your mind which creates a lot of negative emotions? If so, access your playfulness and curiosity, and calm and relaxed state wherein you can think in a more clear-headed way.

> When are you at your best?
> Imagine being there fully and completely right now.
> What is that like? Just notice on the inside... How do you know you are in a centered, focused, and mindful state?
> What is your breathing like, posture, facial expression, tone of voice...

For producing, directing, and editing your new movie you'll need to be able to *step out* of the movie whenever you need to or choose to. Are you able to do that? Practice doing this by stepping into an experience and then stepping out into a state of playful curiosity. Doing this gives you a powerful state or pattern interrupt. It's like all other kinds of interrupts that jar you out of a state of mind and emotion. It temporarily shifts you to another focus and so keeps you in control of your choices. What will you set up as a trigger for your interruption state?

Step 2: Set some awesome frames before you start.
The ability to film a fearful event and to keep it alive in your mind-body system for years, even decades, is actually a pretty amazing achievement, especially when you think about all the things we forget. Recording a film

of fear and terror and being able to step into it so that Steven King is envious is a form of accelerated learning.

Consider the ability to have the hell scared out of you and to then link it to a tone, voice, word, object, event, etc. so that you *never forget* to freak out when you think about that trigger!   That's amazing, don't you think?

Now that you know that your movies affect your emotions, behaviors, response patterns, when you change the movie, it's going to have extensive and pervasive transforming influences throughout your whole mind-body system. Mostly this process will neutralize that old movie so that you'll just eliminate it from your archives of old videos. Is that okay with you?

> Who will you be when you no longer have that particular fearful or traumatizing movie in your head?
> How will this transform your everyday life?
> How will it make a difference tomorrow?

Step 3: Pull out the mental movie that scares you and step out.
What's the fear? What is the phobia about? What strong aversive emotions arise because of it? As you pull out the fear video in your mind, put it upon the screen in your mind and *step out as if you were in a movie theater.*

As you imagine yourself in a movie theater, put the first scene of the movie as a still snapshot up on the screen and get yourself comfortable in a seat in the tenth row. In your mind float to that position and settle down comfortably where you can sit back and watch it. Smell your bag of popcorn or some other special treat, and enjoy getting ready to see it for the last time.

Now with that snapshot on this screen, if there's any color in it, let that fade out until it is just a black-and- white photograph of that younger you. Do you see that younger you? Do you see what that person was wearing? The place where it happened?

Step 4: Step out a second time by floating into the projection booth.
You have now stepped out of the old movie once to observer position. Now you can just observe, just witness the events. To stabilize this, let's do this same process one more time to yet one more level as you float back and up into the projection booth were you can make editorial changes to the movie.

Experience the sensation of the feelings of *floating out of your body* there in the tenth row as you *float back and up* to the projection booth. ... That's right. Float all the way back... until you can see the back of your present day self watching the snapshot on the screen.

And enjoy the feeling of putting your hands on the plexiglass separating you from *the self observing you* in the tenth row watching the snapshot of the younger you on the screen with the full knowledge that a cinematic transformation is shortly about to take place.

From the editor's position you can use your hands at any time to point or gesture at these other locations. You can pantomime the feeling of being behind a protective plexiglass, safe and secure, and able to take full control of the movie and all of its editorial features. And you can feel really safe here because this is the editing room. Here you can edit your films to make them more sane and healthy.

Step 5: Review the fearful cinema for the last time.
Just let the snapshot on the screen become a black-and-white movie and review the old terror or fear or trauma to the end of the show ... Just let it play out and you can let it run as you watch it from here in the projection booth through whatever hurtful, ugly, unpleasant, even traumatic events ... just observing, just watching, and just feeling safe and comfortable *outside* the movie ... because you are no longer in it, but just observing it and so let the scenes play out ... all the way to the end ... and then let it play out a little further until you see to some scene of comfort or pleasure ... Some time after the unpleasant experience when you were with friends and having some fun or relaxing or something like that ...

Now if at any time you feel a pull that invites you to step back into the movie, just *feel the plexiglass in front of you* and know that you can just watch in the safety and protection of this editing room because the movie is about a younger you in another time and place, and you are safe here today.

If at any time you need to have the movie play out more quickly through scenes, do so... you are just observing the events as an onlooker... When the event that was traumatic is over... go to a scene where you're okay, when things are fine. Perhaps you're enjoying a hot bath or shower, a vacation, a party, reading a book, something of comfort and pleasure.

Step 6: Stop.   Intermission Time.

Now after you have come to the scene of comfort, freeze frame that event and stop for a moment. Good. You got through it ... for the last time. In just a moment you are going to do something really weird. An explanation will come later, but for now just listen to the instructions about what to do. When you have a clear sense of the way you're going to play with this old fear movie in your mind, then it will be time to do it.

In just a minute, *step into the comfort scene* or the scene of pleasure at the end of the Movie ... and just be there fully—seeing, hearing, feeling, smelling, tasting through your own eyes, ears, and skin. Stepping into the Movie and being the actor in all of that comfort and pleasure. And be sure to let everything turn into living color. Then, when you're ready, *while inside the movie*—push the fast re-wind button and let it zoom backwards to the beginning of the movie in super fast-rewind so that it takes all of one or two seconds. zooooommmm! And you're *inside the comfort* when this happens ... so that everything goes backwards, including you... Zooming for the beginning black-and-white snapshot.

Ready? Go! ... and zooooommmm! There you go. Good. Alright, interrupt your state ... blow that whistle ... stand on your head ...

Step 7: Play it Again.

Running your movie backwards while you're an actor in the scene of comfort *inside it* from a place of comfort is a strange thing and it takes the brain a little bit to learn this one, so repeat this process five to eight more times.   Each time start at the comfort or pleasure scene and run it backwards. Each time when you step in at the end and rewind all the way back to the first snapshot ... let everything — sounds, sights, feelings, sensations, everything go backwards faster and faster and faster .... It's important to interrupt your state at the end.

As you do, then open your eyes, clear your mental screen. Then, *step into the comfort scene* at the end again, and before you can think about it, do a fast rewind from inside. It's a ride! So blast through it.

How did you like that? Open your eyes. It's over. Good. Let's do that again. *Step into the Comfort scene* again... yes, it's such a bother! But humor me. Okay, are you fully there? Ready for the Super Fast Rewind? Zooooommm.

Step 8: Test to check the results.

After you have run the movie backwards from inside it five to eight times, it's time to test things. We specifically want to find out if you are able any longer to play the old fear movie and get your body full of fright. So try it. See if you can get the old feelings back, whether it was a phobia or just some strong negative emotions. Try really, really hard ... as hard as you can to see if you can get those feelings back.

No? Not as much. Well try harder. Still no? Well, imagine the next time something in your future may trigger it as it has in the past. Try to see if that will get it back.

Drop Down Through Pattern

This pattern involves using the metaphor of *dropping* and/or *falling,* and using that idea and *the feeling of falling* as the frame that you then apply to experience that you want to fall away from. Applying the feeling of falling to an experience is a meta-stating process although now you are applying "dropping down" to the previous state and this shifts the basic meta-state metaphor from going up to going down. Here you will apply *dropping* until you get to the bottom of things—below all of the feelings. Eventually you will get to "the ground," or to a void, and then you will drop below that as well.

The pattern starts with a painful emotional state that you actually feel in your body. When you identify that, you will then drop below that feeling to what was before that. Typically as you drop, you will be dropping into less and less intense states. Then, frames-by-implication, after you pass through the bottom or the ground, you will move into increasingly more positive states. After the third or fifth positive states, one that is powerfullyi positive and valuable to you, you'll use that one to meta-state the first and to "clean the pipes" so to speak.

The Pattern
1) Identify and anchor the feeling of falling.

> Have you ever experienced the feeling of falling?
>
> *Menu list:* Dropping in an elevator, on a roller-coaster, hitting turbulence while in a plane, stepping on something and having it give way under you.

2) *Identify the experience and emotion you want to transform.*

What emotion, feeling, memory, or experience would you like to transform?

Where do you feel it?   What do you feel in your body that dis-empowers you?

How do these emotions or experiences undermine your success?

3) *Step into that experience.*

For the purposes of transformation, recall that experience and step into it so that you see what you saw, hear what you heard, and fully feel what you felt. Be there again. .... Good.

Where do you feel this in your body?

What does it feel like?

How intense are you experiencing this emotion?

Good, just be there with it for a moment, noticing ... just noticing it fully... knowing that it is just an emotion and that you are so much more than any emotion...

4) *Drop down through the experience.*

This may feel strange, but you do know what it feels like when you *drop* ... so feeling that feeling of *dropping*, just drop down through that experience until you drop down underneath that feeling...

What feeling or emotion lies underneath that emotion?

And now just imagine dropping down through that feeling ... [Use the person's language precisely.]

And what feeling comes to you as you imagine yourself dropping down through that one?

[Keep repeating this dropping-down through process until the person comes to "nothing..." That is, to no feelings ... to a void or emptiness.]

5) *Confirm the emptiness.*

Just experience that "nothingness" or "void" for a moment. Good. Now let that nothingness open up beneath you and imagine yourself dropping through and out the other side of the nothingness.

What are you experiencing when you come out the other side of the nothingness? What or whom do you see?   [Repeat this several times .. to a second, third, or fourth resource state.]

6) *Take the positive states and meta-state the first problem state.*

Use each resource state to meta-state each problem state.

And when you feel X about Y, how does that transform things?

And when you even more fully feel X — what other transformations occur?

Valid and solidify: just stay right here in this X resource and as you experience it fully, what happens to the first problem state (#1)?

When you *feel this (*fire anchor for each resource) ... what else happens to those old problem states?

7) *Test.*

Let's see what now happens when you try, and I want you to really try to see if you can get back the problem state that we started with. When you try to do that, what happens?

Do you like this?

8) *Check ecology and future pace.*

Are you fully aligned with this? Any objections to this in the back of your mind?

Would you like to take this into your future?

Into all of your tomorrows and into all your relationships?

Neuro-Semantic Learnings for a Neuro-Semanticist

You are not stuck with your frames or your meanings. You created them, you learned them, you practiced them— and you can destroy them, unlearn them, and stop acting on them. This is your power to create a whole new way of life whenever you want to.

• What frames are still inside you that limit or interfere? Are you now ready to release them?

• What method or methods of deframing do you find that work best for you?

End of Chapter Notes:

1. Meta-Yes Belief Change pattern uses the power of a meta-yes and a meta-no to refuse a belief that you know does not serve you and that creates unnecessary limitations. See that pattern in *Secrets of Personal Mastery* (1997) and in the APG training manual.

2. Anchoring is a basic NLP process whereby you link a trigger to an experience in such a way that now the trigger will set off that experience, especially a felt experience. See *User's Manual of the Brain, Volume I* for a full description. Also, any basic introduction book to NLP will have a description of anchoring.

3. The Movie Rewind pattern in NLP is called by a number of names: Phobia Cure pattern, Visual-Kinesthetic Dissociation pattern, etc. You can find the pattern in *The Sourcebook of Magic* (1997). It is also on the website, www.neurosemantics.com. See the articles on Stuttering, we use this pattern with anyone who has a strong emotional charge to an experience, a charge so strong it is hard to even think about it.

4. At Richard Bandler's request, I wrote a 25-year update of the Meta-Model in 1997. Originally it was to be co-authored, but later that agreement fell apart. The book that was produced is now titled, *Communication Magic* (2001).

5. See the book, *Mind-Lines: Lines for Changing Minds* (1997/ 2005).

"As humans, we are born (and can escalate) a trait that other creatures rarely possess: *the ability to think about our thinking.* We are not only natural philosophers, we can philosophize about our philosophy, reason about our reasoning. ... We can, though we do not have to, observe and judge our own goals, desires, and purposes. We can examine, review, and change them. We can also see and reflect upon our changed ideas, emotions, and doings. And we can change them. And change them again—and again!"

Albert Ellis (1988, pp. 14-15)

Chapter 14

ACTUALIZING CREATIVITY

Creating Meaning and Reframing

"We must become more interested in the creative process, the creative attitude,
the creative person rather then the creative product alone."
Abraham Maslow (1963)

"The problem of creativeness is the problem of the creative person."
Abraham Maslow (1971)

Actualizing your ability for creativity makes real your central powers as a creator of meaning. This means fully owning, acknowledging, and using your powers for creativity and innovation. As a meaning-maker, your most fundamental performance is that of creating meaning. You are an inventor—you invent your reality. Yet how do you do that? By framing, of course! So what skills are required for you to be able to frame the highest and best meanings?

Framing — The Constructing of Meaning
A *frame* is a reference point or reference context. This terminology originates from the idea of a "frame of reference," which we shorten to the single term—*frame*. Framing speaks about an idea, a thought, or a context —*it is a mental context that enables you to understand or interpret*

something.   Suppose when we meet for business conference, I say the following:

> "Hello, glad you showed up. I've only got 25 minutes and then I have to rush to my daughter's school for her play, is that okay? I think we can cover what we need to in that time, do you?"

What frames have I thereby set? I have *set a time* frame (25 minutes), a *reason* for leaving frame (my daughter's play), and a *meaning* frame (do what we need to do), as well as a *collaboration* frame (Is that okay?). These

> The Frames you Create —the Reality You Live

frames present both content (25 minutes, daughter, play, etc.) as well as they set an *interpretative* context for what will thereafter transpire. They enable you to interpret what I thereafter say and do.

If I say, "Hello, how are you?" how do you know how to interpret those words? Here the frame will be set not only with words of greeting by the place, time, and context. If I'm a good friend and we are in a pub, "Hello, how are you?" will mean and be interpreted very different than if you are a client coming in the front door of my psychotherapy office. Or if the words are uttered by a person in a white lab coat in the emergency room.

Framing is the easiest thing in the world to do. Just open your mouth and say words, and with those words you will set some frames. That's because your words come with assumptions and implications. As every word, term, and sentence has both denotation and connotation meanings, every word, term, and sentence not only explicitly convey information, they also implicitly and covertly conveys information about the information. This is meta-information—information about context and how to interpret the words that are uttered.

People who are in the helping professions ask different initial questions when they begin a business conversation.
*   Start is with, "So what's up, what's been happening?" and you will probably invite chit-chat, gossip, and a relaxed low-key atmosphere.
*   Some start conversations by asking, "So what's your problem?" Do this and you implicitly convey the idea (or frame) that problems are important, you are a helper in solving problems, you are inviting a relationship with the person so that you want to explore and solve the person's problems.

- Some start conversations by asking, "So what is the most transformative thing should we talk about that will unleash your potentials?" That's a very different frame. It's a self-actualization frame that assumes that any single conversation may be the most important conversation of your life.

The Art of Setting Frames

So, how do you *set a frame* when you speak, act, and relate? What are the processes by which you and I can become more competent in setting frames for ourselves and with others?

1) State a Singular Core Point

When you use words to set an interpretative context so that you and others will *think in terms of and through that schema,* use words that are direct, clear, focused and that succinctly summarize the essence of your point. If you can do that, you tremendously increase the likelihood of succeeding in setting a frame.

> "How much *fun* do you think you will have in learning at this training?"
> "What would be *the most relevant solutions* to this problem that will enable us to become more efficient and effective?"

What is your core point? What is the one thing that you want to set as the essence of your idea or message? If you don't know it, you obviously will not be able to set it. If you do know it, then practice stating and restating it until you can put it in a single short sentence, or in a phrase, or in a single word. The shorter and tighter you can make the essence of your point— the better. Making your point singular, elegant, and focused like an ad strapline is not easy or quickly done. To do so means to make it semantically loaded with lots of meaning and then to compact it so that it is pregnant with meaning and requires someone to unpack it. When it is that elegant, it has a profound simplicity to it.

2) Ground the Message in the Real World

Knowing your core message is the beginning, once you have that, make sure you ground it. Make it concrete by describing it in sensory-based terms so people can see, hear and feel what you are talking about. If you fail to do this, your words might be elegant, but they will also be abstract and conceptual. So use what writers call "killer details"— ground them in what, where, who, when, how, etc. This will build credibility for the frames you set because it makes them real, actual. This is not "dumbing down," it is connecting with what is real and actual.

As you do this, make sure that you make the facts vividly concrete. Facts do not have to be boring. Consider how any great film director or screen-play writer uses the cinematic features of the everyday facts to make a movie come alive in vivid color and action. This also will boost credibility of the frame and make your invisible point visible to the understanding and perception of your listeners.

3) Set an Engaging Direction
If you want to become truly skilled in *frame setting,* then use words and ideas that set a direction, which create a sense of a desirable future. That is, use language in such a way that it invites people to want to be a part of the world and future that the words indicate.

To do that, reflectively think about the implications of your words and use those that are more appropriate to your mutual purposes. What do my words imply? How might another person take this term or sentence?

> "Are you ready to make a decision or do you need to weigh the pros and cons and be clearer about the price you'll pay in making that decision?"
> "Would you like to focus on clearly identifying the problem and make sure it is well-formed?"

4) Deliver with Emphasis and Energy
You not only set frames by what you say, but also by how you say them. Your tone, speed of speech, tempo, emphasis, etc. all play a role in how another will interpret them. Speak too fast or too slow, or with a certain accent that has certain meanings in a cultural context, and you will set frames for how others will interpret your words. If you want someone to be playfully curious about your idea, then use a voice, accent, or style that conveys playfulness and curiosity. Can you do that? Are you willing to learn how to do that? I like to use Yoda's tone of voice and his curious, "Hmmmmmm" to begin a sentence.

> "Hmmmmmm. Try there is not, only do."

All of this requires that you reflectively consider how you deliver your words. What emphasis and with what energy do you need to put into your delivery so that you can achieve your objectives?

Verbal delivery, other than monotone, inherently involves emphasis. What words do you emphasize as you speak? Where do you put stress? How do you mark out a phrase or word or sentence? How do you put certain words in "quotes." How do you underline ideas that you want to emphasize. If you listen, you will hear semantically loaded terms by how and where a person emphasizes various words. By this you can set a frame. The language pattern described here is "embedded questions or statements," a hypnotic language pattern.[1]

5) *Choreograph Your Semantic Space*

Mind your semantic space and how you work within that space. Beyond the variables of your voice are the variables regarding your gestures, movements, breath, and all of the kinesthetic factors regarding how you move and put energy into your words. Against, this is more about *how* you communicate your words than the content of the words. Semantic space refers to how you tend to externalize on the outside in the space around you in your internal landscape. Where you point to when you refer to the past, the present, and the future makes up the domain of time-lines in NLP. Where you put people refers to your social panorama, another NLP distinction.[2]

In Neuro-Semantics we have taken this further and have identified how people semantically load various gestures and space. You can learn to recognize a person's semantic space by opening your eyes and ears to see and hear what a person is externalizing as they speak. Then you can use that structure as you speak to them. You can use that externalized semantic space to set new frames that will empower them.

6) *Use Repetition to create Refrains*

Repeat your words or sentences. You can *set* a frame by simply repeating a words or sentence, setting it aside and "holding" it as it were so that you or another person can then respond to that rather than racing on to say more words. Doing this allows you to invite the person to move up the ladder of meaning, to scale up through his or her matrix of meanings and so to detect the fuller belief system within which the meaning is embedded. You can establish an idea as a frame by repeating it thereby making it seem more real and present. Perhaps you've noticed that I've done that with the frame,

> "The person is never the problem; if there's a problem, the frame is the problem."

7) *Tease to Evoke Curiosity and Suspense*

Evoke or tease someone with new or challenging possibilities. Frames can also be set by evoking them, even teasing someone to invite them to create a new idea. Here you can use humor or playfulness or you can use challenge and competition. "So what do you think would be the wildest dream that you could come up with about developing this competence of leadership?"

You can't set a frame if you don't get attention. This is always and predictably the first problem of communication—getting attention. So how will you do that? How will you get and maintain the attention and interest of someone? For this, be unpredictable. Obviously, when you become predictable, you also become boring. People know what's coming next and so tune out. So once you have your core message, ask yourself: "What is counter-intuitive about it?" "What is unexpected about this message?" Then use that as how to set a frame that teases thereby evoking curiosity and suspense.

As you do, is there any mystery left in your frame? Make sure there is. If you say it all, then why would anyone keep listening? So don't say it all! Hold back and keep mystery in your message. After all, everybody loves a good mystery story that keeps the suspense going until the end. Otherwise your listeners will get up and leave before the credits.

> "Mysteries are powerful because they create a need for closure. The *Aha!* experience is more satisfying when it is preceded by the *Huh?* experience." (*Made to Stick,* 2007)

8) *Surprise to Shock, Set up the Unexpected and to Create Fascination*

To set a frame that will stick, ask questions and especially bold and surprising questions. Can you set frames by asking questions? Are you aware of how questions direct a mind so that minds go places in search of answers? Did that question set any frames? The best questions are those that delightfully surprise a person. Surprise a person with a question that he or she cannot immediately answer and you almost inevitably send the person on an internal journey to answer the question.

> "So you are highly skilled in procrastination? Would you say that you are at world-class level as a procrastinator? So just to confirm: You have lots of ways to put something important off and then at a later time to regret having put it off? So if you are so good at this, if you were to use this putting-off skill on procrastination itself and

then put off or procrastinate on exercising or anything else that you
know is important, how much would that change things for you?"

By teasing and surprising as you speak, you activate the listener's emotions
so that they stay engaged, become interested, and care about knowing where
you are going or what you are saying. And unless those listening to you are
engaged in this way, they won't *feel* that your message is important or worth
their attention. If emotions get us to act, then what emotion will you seek
to elicit in those you are speaking to? What do you want them to feel?
Getting them to believe is not enough. You have to get them to care—to
feel the importance of the belief.

9) Modify your Words with Dynamic Qualities
Toss in modifiers. If you noticed, I wrote that questions can "delightfully"
surprise. *Delightful*, as a modifier, set an interpretative frame around the
question. This offers a fascinating way to integrate meta-states in your
language without needing to officially or formally meta-state. Now you can
just qualify your statements with the states that you want the person to apply
to a previous state. So if you talk about calm anger or respectful anger, or
playful curiosity, or solid self-esteeming, the qualifiers you use can subtly set
frames in a way that's almost invisible.

10) Formulate as a Gripping Story
I've saved the best for last. Give the essence of your core point a human
face—tell it as a story. You could tell it as a suspenseful story, a mystery,
a drama, etc., but however you tell it— give it the flesh-and-blood realness,
concreteness and power of a story. As a story, your idea then will come
alive, be much more memorable, and can possibly captivate the minds and
hearts of your listeners.

Abraham Lincoln and the Setting of Frames
If "He who sets the frame controls the game" is the principle, then what
Abraham Lincoln did at Gettysburg during the American Civil War with his
speech is a great example.

So what happened at Gettysburg in 1863? A horrible battle and defeat for
the North. The North's general, Meade, had so bungled the battle, leaving
Lee to regroup, that he submitted his resignation to President Lincoln. But
Meade's opponent, Lee, did no better, marching blindly into slaughter—so
great a blunder that he also submitted his resignation.

So those are the facts on the ground: a field of corpses, defeat for the North, disaster, death, civil war. Yet who today remembers Gettysburg that way? No one except perhaps scholars of history. Today Gettysburg is a symbol of heroism as noted by Harry Beckwith (1997):

> "The enormous gulf between the perception of Gettysburg and the reality can be explained in 276 words: the Gettysburg Address. With one deft speech, Lincoln changed almost everything— including our view of the Declaration of Independence and the view of millions of Americans living then and now."

So what happened? Words. The words that set the frames for how to think about and interpret that event, the words that Lincoln set forward in his now famous Gettysburg Address. And it is now those words that continue to govern our memories and perceptions about the battle that occurred so long ago. His words began, "Fourscore and seven years ago ..."

How to Solidify Frames
You can not only set frames, you can also strengthen and solidify a frame so that it sticks— it stays with a person. Since a frame is an interpretative context or scheme by which we view something and understand it, as a mental process, it can become weak and dissolve. To prevent that from happening, you will want to know how to solidify frames.

1) Condition a pattern.
Repeat the frame and set up a trigger (an anchor) so that it is repeatedly triggered. Learning to think with a given frame is most essentially a matter of repetition until it becomes an unconscious mental habit of how to interpret things.

2) Intensify with an emotion.
Bring strong emotion to the frame. The more emotion you bring to a frame, the more that frame becomes attached to that emotion and to the intensity of that emotion. This again is the meta-stating process. Bring joy to your learning, bring curiosity to your confusion, apply respect to your frustration and upset, etc. You can do this directly by eliciting a strong emotional state or you can do this more indirectly by using a story or metaphor.

The Gettysburg Address

Four score and seven years ago our fathers brought forth on this continent, a new nation, conceived in Liberty, and dedicated to the proposition that all men are created equal.

Now we are engaged in a great civil war, testing whether that nation, or any nation so conceived and so dedicated, can long endure. We are met on a great battle-field of that war. We have come to dedicate a portion of that field, as a final resting place for those who here gave their lives that that nation might live. It is altogether fitting and proper that we should do this.

But, in a larger sense, we can not dedicate -- we can not consecrate -- we can not hallow -- this ground. The brave men, living and dead, who struggled here, have consecrated it, far above our poor power to add or detract. The world will little note, nor long remember what we say here, but it can never forget what they did here. It is for us the living, rather, to be dedicated here to the unfinished work which they who fought here have thus far so nobly advanced. It is rather for us to be here dedicated to the great task remaining before us -- that from these honored dead we take increased devotion to that cause for which they gave the last full measure of devotion -- that we here highly resolve that these dead shall not have died in vain -- that this nation, under God, shall have a new birth of freedom -- and that government of the people, by the people, for the people, shall not perish from the earth.

3) *Validate.*
Invite meta-level validating of the frame. Frames are also solidified as they are valued, identified with, and believed in. So simply ask meta-questions to invite this validating. "Do you really want this? Why? What is important about this? And what else? So you really do believe in this? Is this also part of your identity?" To validate more implicitly, apply a value to the frame. Take something that you know is important for you or another person and apply it to the idea.

4) *Provoke.*
Get the person to fight for their frame and experience. "So do you want this?" "You don't sound very convincing, maybe I should take this away from you? Maybe you don't yet deserve this?" When you playfully provoke a person in this way, they will being to fight for their belief frame. They will argue for their frame and that will have the effect of inducing them to more thoroughly incorporate it within themselves. Provocations like this invite the person to access and apply a lot of energy to something and so confirms its value and importance.

5) *Future pace.*
Future pace the person's experience with the frame. In NLP, future pacing refers to getting a person to imagine the future and then—seeing, hearing, and feeling oneself going into that future—experiencing the skill or belief and testing it in that imagined scenario. This enables one to test the experience, to see if it will work out (in the mind), and then perhaps identify other resources to add to the plan.

Meaning takes so many forms. Meaning can take the form of words, perceptions, states, and representations. Given that, there are four meta-domains and meta-models that describe these facets of meaning. Now the tricky thing about this is that rather being four different domains about four different subjects, these four *meta-domains* are four avenues to the same thing—to a subjective experience. And, as four pathways to a singular experience, they give you four descriptions of the same thing.

Reframing for New Creativity
Once you know how to frame meaning, how to de-frame meaning, then re-framing meaning is simply a combination of these two processes. Reframing is creating a new or another frame, a frame that will replace the first one and offer a new one.

As you identify an old meaning that needs to be reframed, first you deframe it. You do this for several reasons. By de-stabilizing the old meaning, you make it less solid and rigid, you move it from being solid to being ambiguous and open to some new and different interpretations. Having done that, another purpose is to identify the various bits and pieces of the old meaning that you can use in the reframing. Deframing takes the experience back to the descriptive level where it can now be framed in many different ways.

And how many ways can you reframe? In *Mind-Lines: Lines for Changing Minds* (1997/ 2007) I took, with Bob Bodenhamer, the original NLP set of distinctions called "Sleight of Mouth" patterns with its 15 ways to shift meaning and reformulated it into the Mind-Lines Model. This model has seven directions and 26 ways to reframe a meaning. By the fifth edition (2007) it was obvious to me that I could extend the reframing to 30 or 50 or 100 more.

What insight led to that awareness? The Meta-State Model awareness that once you have a particular behavior and meanings by which you define that behavior, you can reframe its meaning in as many ways as you can meta-state it with another frame. Every state you bring to it, every frame you bring, every concept, every belief, every understanding, every intention, and so on — has the possibility of reframing.

Seven Directions for Reframing

There are seven directions that you can send a mind in order to shift meaning. With these seven different ways to directionalize consciousness you can re-construct new perspectives, meanings, experiences, emotions, and resources in the reframing:

- Down: we can deconstruct the meanings   — Deframing
- Lateral: we can shift between this and that meaning —   Reframing
- Backward: we can go back in time   — Pre-Framing
- Forward: we can go forward in time   — Post-Framing
- Counter: we can turn the meaning on the person   —   Counter-Framing
- Upward: we can go meta and above the meaning   —   Out-Framing
- Analogously: we can go to the side and create a metaphor or story that is like the meaning   —Analogous Framing

Chart 1
The Mind-Lines Model

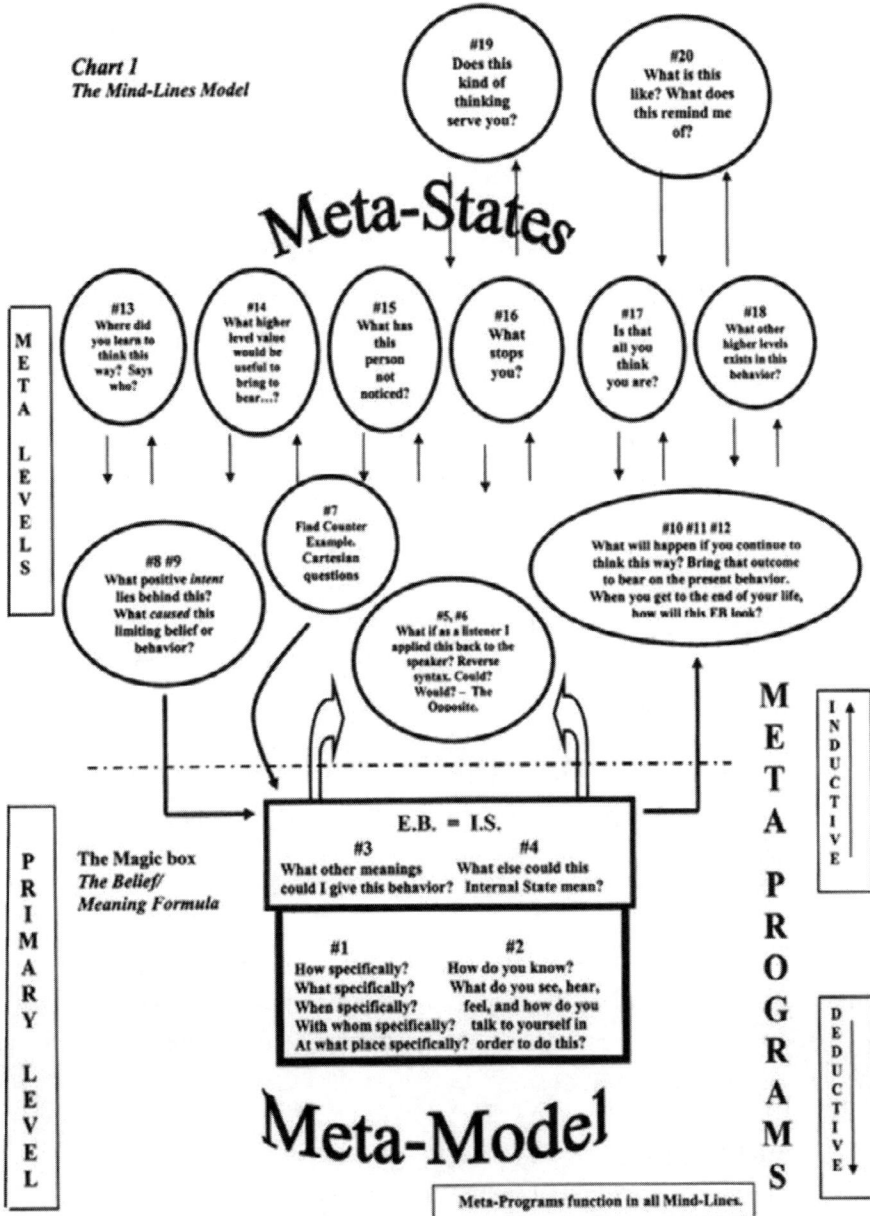

#19
Does this kind of thinking serve you?

#20
What is this like? What does this remind me of?

Meta-States

#13
Where did you learn to think this way? Says who?

#14
What higher level value would be useful to bring to bear...?

#15
What has this person not noticed?

#16
What stops you?

#17
Is that all you think you are?

#18
What other higher levels exists in this behavior?

M E T A   L E V E L S

#7
Find Counter Example. Cartesian questions

#8 #9
What positive *intent* lies behind this? What *caused* this limiting belief or behavior?

#5, #6
What if as a listener I applied this back to the speaker? Reverse syntax. Could? Would? – The Opposite.

#10 #11 #12
What will happen if you continue to think this way? Bring that outcome to bear on the present behavior. When you get to the end of your life, how will this FR look?

The Magic box
The Belief/ Meaning Formula

P R I M A R Y   L E V E L

E.B. = I.S.

#3
What other meanings could I give this behavior?

#4
What else could this Internal State mean?

#1
How specifically?
What specifically?
When specifically?
With whom specifically?
At what place specifically?

#2
How do you know?
What do you see, hear, feel, and how do you talk to yourself in order to do this?

M E T A   P R O G R A M S

I N D U C T I V E

D E D U C T I V E

Meta-Model

Meta-Programs function in all Mind-Lines.

1) Deframing
Take whatever meaning someone offers you (a representation, idea, understanding, belief, reason, excuse, etc.) and embracing it, enter it, analyze it, and identify its component pieces. De-construct its elements and variables.
- How do you know that?
- What are you aware of?
- In what sensory representation are you representing that?
- What else is there? How do you know that?
- How do you link X with Y?
- Where did you learn to think and make sense of things in this way?
- What comes first, second, third, etc. that makes up the sequence?

2) Reframing
From deframing the components and variables, you can see how a meaning is constructed and how to shift that construct. In the Mind-Lines Model, we use the formula of X (an external behavior, EB) leading to ($->$) or equaling ($=$) a Y (an internal state IS). This gives **EB=>IS** as a formula that you can use to analyze meaning and recognize its structure.
- Are you sure that X leads to, or is, Y?
- What if that X was actually something else, a Z? What would that mean to you?
- What's the possibility that X is actually Z?
- Would you like it to be that?
- You know, if you really want to see Y (IS), you ought to take a look at J (EB)!
- It is not X, it is Y.

The meaning equations and attributions of the formula define the neuro-semantic reality for a person, that person's meanings and associations. So the person says, "It means this!" In reframing, you inquire or assert that it means something else.

3) Counter-Framing
When you find the formula of a person's meaning construction, you can now test it by using it on them. That will challenge the belief to see if it equally applies in other situations. If not, it will often just "pop" and vanish. That is, the meaning will not make sense and so implodes. At times, it will not disappear, but will loosen up the old belief. Here you look for an exception to the meaning. Here using reflexivity, you ask, "What do you think of the

belief when you apply it to yourself?" "Is that always true? There's never an exception?

- You can't even think of a time when that's not been true?
- Are there no times when that didn't happen?
- What would have to happen for it not to happen?
- That happens always for everyone at all times and forever will?
- Isn't what you're saying and doing right now doing that very thing you're complaining of!
- Why X to you too!

4) Pre-framing

In pre-framing, you explore (or assert) where a meaning came from and/or why a person would have invented it. Sometimes a person will believe something *and hate* himself for it. Simultaneously, the person may feel condemned or fated to believe it. Then the person may feel guilty for it, ashamed of it, contempt himself, and feel helpless to think anything else. What a mess! Now is the time to use pre-framing as a powerful tool. Preframe *a positive frame* about the belief and where it came so that the person can stop beating herself up for it and release her grip on it. This framing is for pacing and validating the person and enabling the person to gain distance from the limiting and negative belief.

- Given all that you've been through, no wonder you came to believe that!
- I can see the value and benefit of why you constructed that understanding, it was because of A and B.
- That makes lots of sense, I'd come up with that way of thinking also if I had been through that!

5) Post-Framing

When you move to post-framing, you move to disturb, upset, and loosen a meaning by provoking the person with the belief in terms of its consequences. Here you will put those consequences in the person's face in a confrontative way and style. You will hold their face to it until they face up to it! Here you meta-state with *consequential thinking* so the person evaluates the value of a meaning over the longer term as the meaning plays out over time.

- What will this idea get you in the next year?
- What consequences will come of it?
- And when you get those consequences full on, what will that then lead to?

- And what if you live your whole damn life that way, what will that get you?
- You really want to pay all of that price for this idea?

6) Outframing

When you step back from the meaning of a belief system (X—> *and* = *Y*) and move up to set some higher frames about it, you can meta-state it with a great many more other meanings. Here you leave the original meaning alone and qualify it with another perspective.

- Where did you get that idea? Does everybody operate from that idea?
- How ecological is it?
- How does it compare with some of your highest values?
- Does it always work?
- Isn't that just an either/or way of thinking?
- What if you looked at it from a both/and perspective?
- Suppose it just vanished away or become untenable for you?
- What is the system of interactions that it operates within? And what is the context that that is within?
- Is that who you are? Are you going to let that define you?
- What have you decided about this?

7) Analogous framing

This meta-stating is applying metaphorical meanings to a belief. It is using narrative in the form of a story, analogy, or metaphor. And by doing this you can be more subtle, indirect, and less confrontative. And yet within the story you can use any and all of the other reframing patterns.

- That reminds me of a story . . .

The Basic Reframe

Isn't it amazing that we have all of these ways to reframe meaning? As amazing as that is, don't miss the most essential reframe. This is the one where you exchange one meaning for another:

- "It is not that meaning, it is this meaning."
- "Could it mean this rather than that?"

This template enables you to now understand *deframing* as saying, "It does not mean that X at all, when you look at it in detail, that meaning falls apart and you can see that it is a construct and one that doesn't work very well at all." Similarly, by counter-framing you similarly *deframe* the construct. By showing that the X-meaning doesn't hold up and cohere when applied to itself, the X-meaning loses its inner coherency.

All of the *out-framing* (including outframing with time that shows up in the pre- and post-framing) essentially says, "When you temper or qualify the X-meaning with this or that frame, the X-meaning is seen in a very different light. The X-meaning is now seen through the frame and so it deframes it entirely, or qualifies it in such a way that the X is no longer just an X, but an X-qualified meaning. It is not X, it is X-qualified-by-the-higher-frame.

In all reframes, you start with a meaning that's been constructed for some event or experience. "A event means X."

"Rolling the eyes means treating others with contempt."
"Speaking in a strained and harsh tonality means that the person is angry at me and will hurt me."
"Making mistakes is embarrassing; people will think I'm inadequate and incompetent."

Then, you we move to a new meaning or new frame. Assert or ask a question that opens up the possibility that the X-meaning is not the only or the best meaning, that there are other constructions you have give to the A event.

Neuro-Semantic Learnings for a Neuro-Semanticist
There is plasticity to the meaning or meanings that you attribute to any event. Because it is fluid, it can change, evolve, de-evolve, and transform. Meaning isn't set in concrete. Meaning isn't a thing. The meanings that you and I give to events, experiences, words, conversations, people, relationships and a thousand other things, are constructs of the mind and therefore flexibly fluid.

1) Take a belief that you have about something (e.g., exercise, budgeting, making money, taking a risk, confronting someone) and analyze it until you get a formula: $X \longrightarrow Y$ or $X = Y$.

2) Once you have the meaning formula, frame and reframe it until you find a new meaning that creates an empowering belief for you.

End of Chapter Notes
1. A lot of these non-verbal facets of communication are identified in the Milton Model, for a full treatment of that model, see Bandler and Grinder, 1976; Hall and Bodenhamer,

User's Manual of the Brain (1999). We put a lot of emphasis on semantic space in many of the Neuro-Semantics trainings, especially the training of trainers (NSTT) and the licensing of Coaches (Meta-Coaching system).

2. There are models in NLP on the externalization of internal mapping, time-lines is one and the social panorama is another. For treatments on these, see *Time-Line Therapy* (1987 Woodsmall and James), *Adventures in Time* (1997, Hall and Bodenhamer), *The Social Panorama,* Lucas Dirks (1996).

3. The seven directions for "sending a brain" comes from the book: *Mind-Lines: Lines for Changing Minds* (1997/ 2005) which explores this subject in depth.

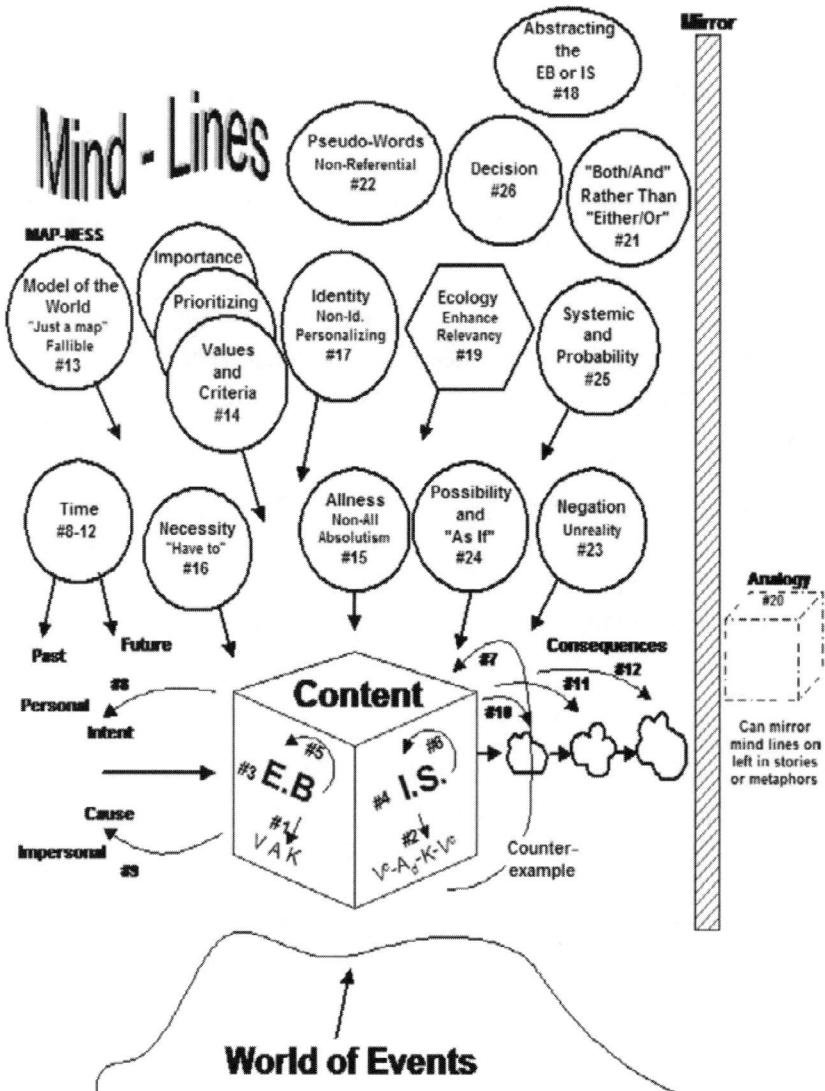

Chapter 15

ACTUALIZING

NARRATIVE MEANING

Inventing New Stories and Metaphors

"Narrative is one of the forms of expressiveness
through which life events are conjoined
into coherent, meaningful, and unified themes."
Donald E. Polkinghorne

"Stories are like flight simulators for the brain."
Chip Heath; Dan Heath (*Made to Stick*)

Narrative meaning arises from an understanding of metaphorical meanings, which we explored in chapter 3. Metaphor, as one kind and representation of meaning, enables the wild and prolific meaning-making that characterizes one of the most creative expressions that we humans are capable of creating. You and I, as meaning-makers, construct meaning by using metaphors and telling stories—indirect and covert methods for the creation of meaning. And when we do this, we are *speaking about one thing in terms of another thing.*

What's a Meta For?

The word *metaphor* literally refers to this wild relationship of speaking about one thing in terms of another. The term "metaphor" itself is informative. Derived from a composite of two Greek words: *meta* (above, about) and *phorine* (to transfer, to carry over) metaphor literally means to "bring one thing over to another thing." When you use a metaphor you invite a listener to create meaningful understanding of something intangible and not easily described in propositional language by comparing it to something concrete or tangible. Aristotle himself said this about metaphors:

> "Metaphor is the application to one thing of the name belonging to another."

When you use a metaphor at a meta-level and/or as a meta-question, the *metaphor* allows you to speak about one thing indirectly by speaking about something more concrete or more familiar. And while all language is metaphorical in nature, when you create or use a metaphor to convey a meaning, you are usually engaged in the creative response of speaking about something vague, intangible, or difficult to describe in terms of something more concrete and well known.

A metaphor is "a figure of speech in which a word or phrase literally denoting one kind of object or idea is used in place of another by way of suggesting a likeness or analogy between them."

Metaphors as the Coding of Meaning

When you look at language at both the level of individual words and statements, metaphors are everywhere. They *lurk in the corners*. They *visit us* like *angels unawares*. At yet other times, you have to *smoke them out*. Most language operates via the structure of metaphors. Metaphor functions as an essential part of how we conceptualize—we compare what we know with what we seek to know and understand.

Lakoff and Johnson (1980a) see metaphor as a basic process for structuring knowledge and constructing meaning. They theorize that concrete conceptual structures form the basis for abstract thinking/talking.

> "We understand experience metaphorically when we use a gestalt from one domain of experience to structure experience in another domain." (p. 230)

In thinking, perceiving, and understanding we constantly find and create metaphors from one experience so that we can then "make sense" of another. In Neuro-Semantics we use metaphors of height and going up to

> The Stories you tell are the Meaning you Live.

understand and experience the idea of expanded awareness and larger perspective. We speak about dragons to understand states that are full of energy and which may devour us. We speak about laser beams to describe the kind of mental focus we desire when we want a strong concentration. We speak about a crucible when we think about a time or place where old structures could melt down and be recasted. And this form of meaning-making with metaphors is a top-down kind of deductive reasoning.

Analogical communication includes metaphors, analogies, similes, stories, and a great many other kinds of figurative language forms. Such language conotates and indirectly implies rather than directly denote a referent. Such language endows communication with less directness, more complexity and vagueness, and typically more emotional evocativeness. It is the language of the poet more than the scientist. I say "more," because scientists also constantly use metaphor. Yet mostly as explanatory devices. Poets, on the other hand, glory in metaphors as an end within itself—for their beauty and charm.

To become sensitive to the metaphorical level and use of language, think in terms of analogies and analogous relations.

> What term, terms, sentences, and even paragraphs imply or suggest some metaphorical relation?
> What metaphors does the speaker use to structure his or her thinking and framing?

What metaphors occur in the following?

> "What you claim is indefensible." "She attacked the weakest point in his line of arguments." "His criticisms were right on target." "They shot down all my arguments."

The overall frame-of-reference here involves conflict, battle, war—these are the driving metaphors here. The speakers analogously compare the communication exchange to soldiers battling to win a war. This greatly differs from another possible metaphor.

"Arguing with him is like a dance." "We danced around the core issue for a long time." "The movements of our meanings whirled around with no pattern at first."

Typically metaphors operate at the level of assumption so that we presuppose the relationship between two things and so experience them unconsciously. This blinds us to their presence and puts them outside of our conscious awareness. So when someone says, "Now I feel like I'm getting somewhere," we may not even notice the "travel" metaphor of journeying and adventuring. "That was over my head" suggests a "space" metaphor to ideas and understandings.

Performing Meaning Construction Via Metaphors

When you use a metaphor to refer to something, you create a rich code with explicit and implicit meanings. What is most obvious are the overt meanings that occur when you denote something. At a less conscious level, there are always covert meanings, connotations that come along with the metaphor. Mark Johnson and George Lakoff calls these "entailments." These are the ideas and feelings that come along with the metaphor that you didn't intend and probably do not want.

From this understanding of the nature of metaphors, two NLP trainers and writers, James Lawley and Penny Thompkins, have developed *Metaphors in Mind: Symbolic Modeling and Clean Language*. They did this by modeling the work of David Grove and how he handled the metaphors that he could in the language of his clients. The focus on modeling the metaphorical landscape of a client is to expand awareness and understanding of the client's model of the world.[1]

Narrative Meaning

An even richer complex of meaning are those that are coded as *narratives* —stories, dramas, case histories, fairy tales, etc. Here meaning is not just a statement or a comparison. Meaning here lives within a full world of premises. Yet these are usually not even noticed due to the seduction of the story itself. And if covert connotations come along with metaphors, they dominate even more and unconsciously with narrative accounts.

Narrative provides a fundamental scheme by which you are able to link individual actions and events into interrelated aspects of an understandable composite— a story. Narrative enables you to connect things to construct larger level meanings. Story allows you to configure events and to hold them together in a scheme which gives cohesion to life. Among the key organizing operations of story or narrative is plot. A plot provides a theme or motif and so sequences actions over time giving your life a sense of direction as you reach forward to important goals. The plot is a larger level frame that holds the events together in a meaningful structure.

Polkinghorne (1988) describes story as a way to configure a set of actions so that they lead to new meanings. As such narrative creates meaning giving life a coherent structure:

"... narrative is a scheme by means of which human beings give meaning to their experience of temporality and personal actions. Narrative meaning functions to give form to the understanding of the purpose of life and to join everyday actions and events into episodic units. It provides a framework for understanding the past events of one's life and for planning future actions." (p. 11)

"Being human is more a type of meaning-generating activity than a kind of object. It is an incarnated or embodied making of meaning— that is, it is primarily an expressive form of being." Narrative is one of the forms of expressiveness through which life events are conjoined into coherent, meaningful, unified themes." (p. 126)

What are the stories that you can use to construct meaning? What are your favorite stories or types of stories? Stories come in many different forms:

Fairy Tales	Movies	Novels
Myths	Horror	Romance
Drama	Melodrama	Comedy
History	Comic strip	Epics

In narratives the basic story-plot comes in terms of a protagonist, a goal, and the kind of change experienced in the process of going after the goal. What happens to the protagonist in relation to a goal that he or she sets? Does the narrative tell a story of progression, regression, and/or stability?

The very act of telling a story enables you to create a causal nexus. That is, you create *a cause-effect story* that explains what an event leads to or what caused some other set of events to transpire. Here, unconscious structures about causation and consequences are built into the structure of the story, a structure so implicit that it is just assumed and therefore not questioned.

> Narrative creates meaning; it enables us to view life a coherent structure.

Then there are "what if" stories or scenarios. We play these out in our heads as we anticipate the future and we often use them to embolden ourselves to move forward or scare ourselves from taking action.

When I say that a narrative "structures" the events of our lives, I'm not referring to a static structure at all. Narrative structuring is dynamic and living so that it is continually evolving and transforming. That means you often able to re-describe a first event afresh in terms of a second event. [This X anticipates, begins, proceeds, provokes, give rise to this Y.] The stories themselves are continuously changing. And those who tell the stories are forever configuring and reconfiguring the narratives, changing them as they learn more and experience more. Stories are wonderful in this way, they live and breath, they grow and evolve.

In your stories about yourself, you are both the storyteller and the audience. Lisnek (1996) has noted the "story" nature of communication and the Meta-Model as a technology for addressing such.

> "There is a term that applies to the story-telling model of communication — it's the 'meta' model. In simple terms, the meta model is based on the idea that people relate information in story form. As listeners of the story, we add to the information we hear or delete facts or impressions based on past experience and our interpretation of events. So, your version will assuredly be different from mine, even if we've both experienced the same event. (pp. 33-34).
>
> "When Arnie tells his best friend Mary about his rotten salary, he tells a story. ... The meta model of communication includes a set of patterns that allows us to examine how we generalize, distort, specify, or delete data as we relate information in our stories. We do this so that we can better position ourselves in negotiation by testing the stories of the other negotiator." (p. 34)

Developing Your Narrative Competence

As with other forms of meaning-making, there is a skill in being able to detect, create, suspend, and change narratives. Do you know *how to story* events, people, statements? The art of narrative consists of putting events into stories in such a way that you make the experience of your life meaningful.

Narrative competence also includes handling and dealing with time as the temporal dimension. So when you plot a story over time, you endow it with a sense of direction. That's because via narrative we order human temporality. About narrative competence, Polkinghorne (1988) wrote:

> "His [Vladimir Propp] structural analysis began with the assumption that the recognition of meaning in a fairy tale is similar to the recognition of meaning in a sentence. As humans have the capacity to detect when a group of words do not cohere into a meaningful sentence, they also have the capacity to detect when a group of narrative sentences do not cohere into a meaningful story." (p. 83)

From this understanding we can now ask several questions about the power of narrative-story to create frameworks of meaning:

- Does the story cohere? Does it account for all of the events and does it hold together as a cohesive whole?
- What is the nature of your stories? Are they liberating or tyrannizing? Toxic or benevolent, conspiracy driven, game show, helpful, etc.?
- How will you finish the story to complete it and give it closure?
- How will you contextualize an event to the story?
- How does the story predict actions, events as the narrative unfolds?
- How well are you able to recognize acceptable / unacceptable stories in a culture?
- Are you able to see the whole, the larger configuration of the narrative?
- Are you able to listen empathically to a story and let the story be told?
- And because behind every story is another story, a larger frame, a meta-story, your cultural story—What is the racial story of your family or nationality? What stories were you born into?

Narrative Creation and Performance Pattern[2]

As story is a mechanism of meaning-making, it operates as a larger frame, one that holds the meanings that you have constructed in place so that *you can then perform that new story by embodying it and enacting it.* The design of the following pattern is to use the narrative point of view to think about and conceptualize your life and then open up space for a new story to develop and to redesign it more meaningfully.

In the field of Narrative Therapy, Michael White (1991) invites people to search for "unique outcomes" in their stories. These *unique outcomes* are the actions or thoughts that do not fit with the dominant or the problem story. The invitation is to find and develop flukes, exceptions, miracles, luck, experiments, surprises, weird events, sparkling events, the unexplained, and the unnoticed as essential to the process of narrating a new story.

> Narrative structuring is dynamic and living so that it is continually evolving and transforming. That means you often able to re-describe a first event afresh in terms of a second event.

Bruner notes that every story has landscapes within which the narrative occurs. There are two landscapes: the landscape of consciousness and the landscape of action. Given this, you can now use each set of questions about each landscape to develop the new story.

Narrative Awareness Pattern
1) Identify an old story and de-construct it.
If your life is a "story," what is the story that you have been born into in your family, culture, country, etc.?
To what extent is your story problem-saturated?
To what extent is it solution focused?
What story or stories have been told and what stories have you told yourself about your life?
When you quality control your story, how useful, enhancing, and empowering is it?

2) Create a new and preferred story.
Identify the story that you desire.
What values does the new story highlight?
What abilities are required by the new story?

Who will you become in the new story?
How will you language the new story?
How will you elaborate the story?
The landscape of consciousness questions ask about intentions, goals, understandings, values, etc. the landscape of action asks about what you will be doing, when, where, with whom, etc.?

What possibilities occurred at previous times of your life that you could now recover and use in a new way — in a way that you have not, so that as you fetch back that possibility, you now make it come alive in a new way?

3) Recruit an audience for your new story.

Who do you want as your audience?
Who will you tell your unfolding story to?
How will you perform the new meaning for your peers, colleagues, family?

4) Practice embodying the story until it becomes lived.

How will you live the new story in your actions?
What actions will you embody and enact that will indicate the new narrative?
How will you tell and re-tell yourself and others this new story until it will habituate and shape your perceptions and behaviors?

Linguistic Time-Lining Pattern
1) Discover your story.

What story have you lived in up until now?
Who storied you with that story?
Is it part of your cultural story, racial story, religious story, family story, etc.?
How much of the story did you personally buy or create?
Tell about the theme of your life and listen to your narrative story.
What kind of narrating do you do?
Do you tell a story of victimhood or survival, of failing or winning, of connecting or disconnecting, of being loved or rejected, etc.?
Since personality arises from our use of "time," and since narrative tends to operate as a large-level linguistic structure that guards "time" and structures "time" (the events we've experienced), we invite you to explore your "time" narratives.

Use one of the following *sentence stems* and generate 5 to 10 sentence completions. This invites you to generate some of your current and operational linguistic time-lining "programs."

A) *Up until now the story of my life has comprised a story of ...*"
[Prompters include: a victim, a failure, bad luck, stress, rejection, ease, success, liked by lots of people, etc.]

B) *If I described the plot that the narrative of my life has enacted....*
     [A tragedy, a drama, a soap-opera, the lone ranger, etc.]

C) Say aloud, *Up until now... I have thought, believed, felt, acted....*
     Then fully describe and express what has characterized some facet of how you have responded mentally, conceptually, emotionally, verbally, behaviorally, etc.

2) *Quality Control.*

Step aside from the story for an expansive meta-awareness that allows you to check the ecology, then evaluate the usefulness, productivity, value, emotional enjoyment, etc. of your story.
Would you recommend living in that story to anyone else?
How well has this narrative served you?
What doesn't work very well or feel very well about that story?
Do you need *a new narrative*?
Do you feel stuck simply because you do not know of *anything else* that you could possibly say about your experiences than what you have already said?
Go *above* time so that you can think *about* the days of your life from there and recode the happenings that occurred *in* time, sometimes prior to "the time" and from "within" the time.

3) *Make up a new story that would be more empowering.*

Once you have identified the "past" linguistically in this way, then complete the statement:
     "But from this day on... I will increasingly develop into more of a person who...
Just for fun, make up a wild and woolly story. Use your "pretender" skill to its fullest capacity! What positive and bright "sparkling moments" have you experienced that has not fit into your dominant story?

What unique outcomes that seem at odds with your problem-saturated story would you have liked to have grown into your dominant story?

How would that have played out?

What story would you have wished to have lived?

Who do you know that you admire and appreciate?

What story do they tell themselves about their self, others, the world, etc.?

4) *Externalize the old story to de-frame it.*

Narrative Therapy's social constructionism highlights that our stories are constructions that we have built and *internalized*. We have internalized the messages offered by our culture, family, and friends. We have taken experiences, problems, emotions, etc. and told a story that went, "I am X..." In NLP, *internalizing* shows up linguistically as nominalizations and identifications.

Now it's time to *externalize* what we have internalized. We can now tell *externalizing stories* to de-construct the old narrative. This separate person and behavior.

> *"The Mads* have had a long history in sneaking up and tempting me to give way to them."

> "Yes, *Misunderstanding* has lured us into treating each other as enemies, but now that we have turned the light on Misunderstanding, we have caught many of its tricks."

Think of a "problem" that you have experienced frequently (an emotion, behavior, circumstance, linguistic label) and externalize it.

5) *Counter-example the unstoried to create a new narrative.*

Finding the un-storied nrrative in your life (i.e., *counter-examples*). Find *exceptions.* Find *unique outcomes* that identify "sparkling events" to seed a new narrative. Ask *how questions.* "How did you do that?"

> How did you not fall into self-pity, but just kept at it?

> How did you resist losing your cool, and listened to your boss anyway?

> How did you not discount yourself in that instance?

> How did you prevent things from getting even worse with all of that happening?

6) Step into the new story to thicken its plot.

Via your imagination, fully and completely step into the re-story and experience it fully in all of the sensory systems. Anchor it. Enrich it with details and find audiences to perform it before.

Telling a new story isn't enough. We have to *thicken the plot.* To do that use questions about sequences of behaviors to *link the past, present, and future together* and to thereby create a narrative of drama and action. Ask questions that presuppose a set of enhancing responses which will enable people in re-narrating their life.

"*How long* have you cared about improving yourself and making a significant contribution? *Have you had any times* when you felt that way? *Why* did you choose to prefer to live your life that way?"

The first question identifies the resource, the second question invites the person to access historical events, the third encourages them to justify, explain, and build up semantic reasons for it. Such questioning encourages people to "thicken the plot" of their preferred life's plot (Freedman and Combs, 1996).

Future pace: imagine moving out into tomorrow living out that story...

Neuro-Semantic Learnings for a Neuro-Semanticist

Meaning-making isn't only about creating conscious propositions. Most of your meaning-making is much more dynamic, dramatic, rich and colorful than merely declaring that one event or experience (X) equals some idea or understanding (Y). Most of your meaning-making is much less disciplined, you simple compare one thing with another and presto—you create metaphoric or narrative meaning.

- What are your key or central metaphors? Go on a search to detect them. Appoint several people in your life to be on "metaphor alert" when you speak.

This makes metaphors and narrative meanings much more covert, implicit, and unconscious as meanings and therefore more outside of your control. It is outside, that is, until you become conscious of it.

- Use the two patterns in this chapter to explore and expand the metaphors that you use in formulating meanings in your life.

End of Chapter Notes

1. See the book, *Symbolic Modeling and Clean Language.* There are the nine basic Clean Questions in Symbolic Modeling:

> And is there anything else about X (the client's metaphor)?
> And what kind of X is that?
> And that X is like what?
> And where is X?
> And whereabouts X?
> And then what happens?
> And what happens next?
> And what happens just before X?
> And where could X come from?

2. The Linguistic Time-Lining pattern comes from *The Source Book Volume II* (2004).

Chapter 16

ACTUALIZING

COMMUNICATION

EXCELLENCE

"Conversations have to be different from what clients are used to
in order to bring about change..."
Gregory Bateson

"We are *in* language,
and that by being in language, we are in activity."
Wittgenstein

Y ou may have noticed in all of the previous chapters that *the process of creating meaning is synonymous with communication.* Your first communication is to yourself as you are thinking, linking, associating, imagining, framing, evaluating, and all of the other things that you do in your mind to construct meaning. Then you communicate the meanings that you hold in your mind to others via speaking, asserting, questioning, telling stories, reporting events, making evaluations, presupposing, requesting, promising, wondering, and all of the other things that you do as you make yourself known to others.

No wonder then that *communication* lies at the heart of Neuro-Semantics NLP. No wonder the field of NLP arose as a communication model and that, as its most essential core, it *is* a Communication Model.   After all, the first NLP Model was a model of the linguistic patterns of three world-class communicators (Fritz Perls, Virginia Satir, and Milton Erickson)— the Meta-Model of Language.

Given this essential role of communication in Neuro-Semantics, it should be no surprise that one of the things that we focus a lot of our attention on is *actualizing communication excellence.*   To that end, most of the basic premises in NLP and Neuro-Semantics are about communication.   To summarize them, I have collected the following twelve statements as core principles of communication.   If you learn and integrate these communication premises, if you let them govern your communications, you will become a professional communicator.

Communication Premises[1]
> 1) Speaking and acting are the key variables in communicating meaning to ourselves and others.
> 2) Communication is *a communion* of understandings between persons.
> 3) We communicate from state to state.
> 4) Communication effectiveness requires rapport — abundant rapport.
> 5) Resistance indicates inadequate rapport, always makes sense, and can be used to facilitate effective communication.
> 6) Communication is negotiated; it is a dance of exploration of messages sent and received, the exchanging of meanings.
> 7) All communication is filtered by meanings.
> 8) The meaning of your communication is the response that you get.
> 9) You never know what you have communicated until you explore the responses that you get.
> 10) Calibrating to the responses that you get gives you clues about the meanings that others have created from your words and non-verbal expressions.
> 11) Communication is always layered with the unspoken thoughts in the back of the mind.
> 12) Communication is psycho-logical.

The Art of Conversational Framing

Wittgenstein (1958) points out that the meaning of words is determined by how they are used as we engage in a conversation in a specific context. *By themselves the words are inadequate to determine the meaning.* The question is *how* I am using the words and *how* you are responding to them. Then out of the interactions we negotiate how we are using the words in our exchanges. And all of this means something very unique: *Meaning is negotiated in conversation.* That's why I can only know what a word means by how those in a conversation are using it. That's why every meaning needs to be indexed to the conversations in which they arise— when, where, with whom, for what purpose?

In Wittgenstein's terminology, such conversations are "language games." That is, it is an activity or "game" between two or more persons as they seek to communicate their ideas, beliefs, understandings, goals, etc. and negotiate with each other using the words that they do as symbols for their inner referents. Austin (1955) talked about this in terms of "the performative role of words" in his classic William James Lecture at Harvard, *How to do Things with Words.*

> "To say something is to do something, or in saying something we do something." (1955, p. 108)

Church (1961) took this idea further:

> "Words do not have meanings, but functions. The 'meanings' assigned to words by dictionaries are abstractions drawn from the way words function in various contexts." (p. 217)

There are so many things that you can do with words! Do you know about all of these things? Here's a short list of critical things you can do with words:[1]

Gather information	Learn something new
Understand someone's perspective	Inform someone of an idea
Seek clarification when confused	Influence people
Bond or connect with someone	De-hypnotize old trances
Express endearment to someone	Validate or affirm someone
Reinforce a behavior or response	Advocate a position
Extinguish an action or response	Define and/or solve a problem
Experience a catharsis of emotion	Apologize for creating a hurt
Confess a fault or problem	Negotiate a new arrangement
Take responsibility for self	Confuse others
Hypnotize self or others	Insinuate something negative
Engage and absorb attention	Swear, offend, and insult

Disclose a secret	Show off
Soothe, nourish, and comfort	Make fun of someone
Create jokes and humor	Expression intentions
Meta-Communicate	Make a declaration
Promise, set an expectation	Adjust a promise

1) Speaking and acting are the key variables in communicating meaning to ourselves and to others.

While it is easy to speak and act, to truly *communicate* is much more difficult. Speaking by itself is not communication; nor is acting. Communication involves so much more—it is a communion between persons—two persons having a communion around some meaning and therefore a "union" with ("co-") each other.

To communicate with each other, you speak words and act in doing things so as to "say" something to the other person. Yet the words and actions do not mean, they are the vessels and symbols that you use to communicate your messages. *Meaning is in you.* Meaning is always in the person and never in the words or the non-verbals a person uses. That's why knowing what you said and how you said it is insufficient to identify what you communicated. More is needed. Yet it all begins here and this demystifies "communication" as it gives you two key variables in how to improve your you communication skills.

2) Communication is a communion of understandings between persons.

The first task of communication is understanding, not agreement. We communicate first to understand each other, what the other person is thinking, feeling, wanting, and doing. As such, to "understand" does not require that you agree, only that you *recognize* what the other person is perceiving and feeling and that we are able to *acknowledge* those thoughts and feelings. Interestingly enough, the word "under-stand" speaks about *standing under* another person, a beautiful picture of supporting another person as a person, as a human being whether you argue with the person about some particular content.

You have reached the first stage of communication when you are able to repeat what the other person is thinking, feeling, believing, wanting, etc. —to his or her satisfaction. If you cannot do that, then you do not yet even *understand* the other person. This is the first thing to negotiate in any communication— if you don't succeed in negotiating that you are first and foremost seeking to understand the person on his or her own terms, the rest of your brilliant communications will mean nothing.

> *By themselves the words are inadequate to determine the meaning.* The question is *how* I am using the words and *how* you are responding to them.

3) We communicate from state to state.

No communication is pure or clean. Whenever you communicate, you are in a state and you communicate from that state to the state of the other person. This seriously complicates communications. The state that you are in causes your communications to be filtered and influenced by your mental-emotional-physical state and it causes your communications to be further filtered and complicated by the state and states of the other person. Your state and the state of others create the emotional context of the exchange and you feel it. We all do. We pick up on each other's moods and attitudes.

That both you and the other person are in some state raises lots of questions which affect the entire communication endeavor:

> What state are you in? What state is the other person in?
> Are these states helpful or useful for communicating?
> How much do that influence the messages that you are attempting to send to the other person?
> Do you need to shift or change your state?
> Do you need to help the other person change his or her state?

How well do you negotiate this aspect of communication? Are you even aware of your state as you begin to speak? What will you need to do to raise your consciousness to this level?

4) Communication effectiveness requires rapport— abundant rapport.

Given that you are always in a state and that your state influences the state of the other person, always begin by matching the other person, seeking first to understand that person, and to create as much rapport with the other person as you can. Effective communication requires the "rapport" of connection, of trust, of a good attitude, of feeling that the other person is trying to be helpful and not hurtful, that the other person cares and is compassionate, etc.

Rapport, as a sense of connection and trust with another person, is what allows the communication to proceed beyond the shallow level of polite exchanges. Rapport enables you to open yourself up to another, and it makes it safe for the other to similarly open up to you. Without rapport, there will be less patience, tolerance, and more reactivity and defensiveness. When there is the lack of rapport, there will be resistance and defensiveness. Without rapport, communication becomes harder to increasingly achieve. You increase your communication effectiveness as you get into a state of rapport with the person (or persons) you want to communicate with.

The structure of rapport is *being like* the other. It is *matching* what they say, their tone, volume, breathing, posture, etc. Observe the external outputs of the other person and then replicate them. That is the easiest way to begin to learn how to pace the other person and to create rapport. Match the other's posture, energy, volume, tone, etc. So are you ready to negotiate a matching of the person or persons that you want to communicate with?

5) Resistance indicates inadequate rapport, it always makes sense, and can be used to facilitate more effective communication.

If you get resistance and do not understand it, then remember: *It always makes sense to the other person and almost always comes from the lack of rapport.* We all resist what feels threatening, disrespectful, or disconnecting to us. We resist when we don't think the other person understands us or cares about us. Resistance always makes sense because it is a way that we protect ourselves against another's intrusions. Resistance is a person's safety mechanism.

What explains this? Trust and vulnerability. If I'm going to trust you—trust that you will not be hurtful, I need to trust that you will be respectful and caring. Letting you in, lets you see my vulnerabilities so I need some evidence that you are trustworthy—that you have the character and ethics to handle the intimacy of connection. People have to earn the right to be allowed entrance. So I look to see if you are respectful, if you are treating people well. The premise is: "Treat someone badly and you will not be let in." So to get entry, enter with respect and care. And this, of course, is the next thing to negotiate.

6) Communication is negotiated; it is a dance of exploration of the messages sent and received —an exchange of messages.

In communicating we send and receive messages. By means of the exchange, we come to an understanding of each other, so that each understands what the other person thinks, feels, and wants. It is in this way that communication is negotiated between two people. We negotiate what we

> *Resistance always makes sense to the other person and almost always comes from the lack of rapport.*

understand with what the other person understands as our messages are sent and received back and forth until a mutual understanding is attained. At that point, we can begin to negotiate what each person wants and how we can attain a frame of agreement so that we can do business with each other. This is as true for negotiating personal relationships as it is for business relationships.

In communication we all bring lots of understandings, interpretations, beliefs, values, and experiences as we exchange these meanings. We do so to seek to understand and to work out some form of negotiation or relationship. Messages sent is more than not—*not* the message received so we have to check, and check again until a state of understanding is created.

7) All communication is filtered by meanings.

The first contamination of our communications is created by the very state or states you are in. Yet it doesn't end there. All of the communications to and from another person are also contaminated as they are filtered by the meanings of your words, understandings, beliefs, values, histories, etc. *No communication is pure or clean.* All communication is contaminated by multitudes and layers of meanings that all of us bring to the exchange of messages.

Expect that in every communication, you and the other is already starting with certain meanings and understandings. In doing that, you start from the premise that you are more likely to misunderstand each other than understand. This is actually the work of communication— to clear out what we do *not* mean so that we can more clearly say what we do mean.

8) The meaning of your communication is the response that you get.

What something means to the person with whom you are communicating depends on how that person responds. That person's response is not only a function of the messages that you send, you words, tones, gestures, breathing, etc., but also all of the meanings that that person brings to the exchange. What your communication therefore means to the other person depends on what the other person hears, understands, believes, values, etc. And so the person's responses give evidence of what your words and non-verbals must mean to him or her.

The meaning of your communication to the other is not what it means to you or what you intend to communicate. The meaning to the other person is what it means to him or her. That's why you never know what you have communicated! That's why we have to notice and ask the other person if you want to find out.

9) You never know what you have communicated until you explore the responses that you get.

Given that the meaning of your communication is the response you get, then you never know what you've communicated! What did you communicate? That's an unknown. It is unknown until you get a response. You can know what you said, how you said it, the tone you used, your volume, your facial expressions, and dozens of other non-verbal expressions. You can video-tape all of that, but still you do not know what you have communicated. That depends on what the person takes and understands from your messages. And that as a way of finding out what the other person *heard,* is the key to communication effectiveness. Now the exploration can begin.

10) Calibrating to the responses that you get gives you clues about the meanings that others have created from your words and non-verbal expressions.

If the other person's responses give you cues and clues about the meanings that he or she is making from your words and non-verbals, then your skill of noticing, hearing, and calibrating to those responses is the foundation for your skill for adjusting your messages. Calibrating refers to your sensory awareness of noticing the responses of the other person. It refers to noticing changes in the other person's responses especially to the non-verbal portions of the messages.

You need feedback from the other person. The other's feedback is information about what he or she has heard and what your words and non-verbal expressions *means* to that person. Without feedback, you won't know what worked and what didn't work, what the person is responding to or reacting to and therefore you won't know what to adjust to get through to that person.

11) Communication is always layered with the unspoken thoughts in the back of the mind.

> The meaning of your communication is the response you get. That's why you never know what you have communicated! And why you have to check it out.

The self-reflexive nature of the human mind truly complicates communication because there are always additional thoughts in the back of the mind about whatever we are thinking and talking about. The first levels of these in-the-back-of-the-mind-thoughts are typically conscious, you are probably aware of what you are thinking but not saying. But after that, the in-the-back-of-the-mind-thoughts are less and less conscious and eventually completely unconscious. The thoughts in the back of your mind are your unconscious thoughts and emotions that make up your frame of mind, your premises, and assumptions.

That's why exploring your unconscious layers of states (thoughts-and-feelings) via meta-questions provides you a way to discover your own Matrix of Frames and well as a tool for discovering those of another.

12) Communication is psycho-logical, the meanings are meaningful from the inside-out.

You never know what something you have said or done means to another person because the *meanings* that he or she gives to your words and actions depend on their internal dictionary and lexicon. Meaning is an inside job in several ways. It is created on the inside by each person and only comes to be shared and mutual through the process of the exchanging of messages.

Neuro-Semantic Learnings for a Neuro-Semanticist

Will the conversation you have today be a life-changing one? Mind-renewing conversation? Any conversation could be. Are you prepared for that? Susan Scott (2002, 2009) has written:

> "The conversation *is* the relationship, and while no single conversation is guaranteed to change the trajectory of a career, a company, a relationship, or a life, any single conversation can."

> 1) Take each of the twelve premises and spend a day using it to guide and direct your own communications. Notice the changes it

creates and how it can empower and enhance your own communication excellence.

2) Since it takes two to communicate, which of the twelve premises would make the most transformative difference in your life as you begin to actualize communication excellence for yourself so you become a professional communicator?

End of the Chapter Note
1. These are part of the NLP presuppositions, the set of premises that hold the theory of NLP in place. You can find various lists of the NLP presuppositions in different books.

2. See *Communication Magic* (2001, pages viii and ix).

Chapter 17

ACTUALIZING

EXCELLENCE

Modeling Experiences of Excellence

"Excellence is never an accident."

"All things excellent are as difficult as they are rare."

When you, or anyone else, actualize your highest and best—what results is *an expression of human excellence.* And that expression of excellence has a structure. That is, there is rhyme and reason for its expression, how it operates, and what makes it appear as it does. Whatever the person is doing to manifest his highest and best, that expression is being made real in the world in an actual form. And for that person, the expression is meaningful and significant.

So if we then explore how it works, detail the specifics of that expression, we can then make explicit its structure or form. And then, with a full description of the person's performance of excellence, we will understand what the person does internally and externally to create it. And that then gives us a map for replicating that excellence. We call this process of identifying, detail, describing, and replicating excellence *modeling*.

Now *modeling excellence* or best practices did not start with Bandler and Grinder when they modeled the three world-class communicators— Fritz Perls, Virginia Satir, and Milton Erickson. A long time before the 1970s when that modeling occurred and launched NLP, Abraham Maslow began modeling Max Wertheimer (co-founder of Gestalt Psychology) and Ruth Benedict (founder of cultural anthropology). That was 1937. That's when he discovered two self-actualizing people and began his "good humans studies." Eventually that expanded to hundreds and then thousands of case studies of self-actualizing people. And from that arose his studies in Self-Actualization Psychology which led to Humanistic Psychology as the "Third Force" in Psychology, the first Human Potential Movement, and his classical books.[1]

The NLP Adventure of Modeling Excellence

Another instance of discovering some amazing people with fabulous skills began when Richard Bandler accidently began to mimic Fritz Perls and discovered that he could recreate Perl's results. Merely copying Perl's words, gestures, and patterns, the "magic" of transformation began occurring. How was that possible? What explained it?

Now one of the most amazing things about NLP modeling is that Bandler and Grinder were actually able to model *the structure of communication excellence* in Perls and Satir using Transformational Grammar. If there was a miracle in the origin of NLP—this is it! Have you ever read Transformational Grammar (T.G.)? Boring! Snore city. And yet, surprise of surprise—they used the distinctions within T.G. to sort out the structure of what was happening in their communications that generated the incredible results. They took the model that Norm Chomsky used to defeat the Behaviorism of Skinner (1956) and created a model of 11-distinctions, the Meta-Model of Language, that allowed them to be able to replicate the communication excellence in two world-class therapists.

And by the way, after they created *The Meta-Model of Language* in 1975-1976, Chomsky refuted and rejected his own model of Transformational Grammar as inadequate and too unwielding to explain linguistics. That was 1976. And by the way also, after the NLP co-founders put a short explanation of Transformational Grammar as an Appendix to the first two NLP books, *The Structure of Magic* (1975, 1976), neither they nor any other NLP writers or trainers ever presented that Appendix or any other extensive description of Transformational Grammar again.

Why not? Because they didn't need it. All they needed were two things. First, the eleven linguistic distinctions which were mostly in the Cognitive Psychology models as developed by Aaron Beck and Albert Ellis and in General Semantics with Korzybski's linguistic distinctions. Second, the idea of levels. And again, we have levels in the meta-level distinctions of Bateson, in Korzybski, and in the Meta-States Model.

NLP Modeling

With the creation of the first NLP Model, the Meta-Model, now they had a tool (a linguistic tool) whereby they could model almost any subjective experience. And that's what Bandler and Grinder, along with the early NLP group of experimenters, started doing—identifying the structure of experiences—how they work and how to refine them.

Soon, however, they developed other tools for modeling. Taking the TOTE model of the Cognitive Psychologists (George Miller, Karl Pribram, and Eugene Gallanter), the early NLP people completed it with the representational systems and lo, and behold— The Strategy Model for modeling.[2]

At the same time, using the representational systems (visual, auditory, kinesthetic) as the "languages of thought" another model was created. It was called Pragmagraphics at first and then changed to Sub-Modalities so it would be simpler.[3] This model refers to the cinematic features that a person can use to code and re-code one's internal representations for thinking about or mapping out an experience. These cinematic features of one's representations actually operate at a higher or meta-level and so, more accurately, are Meta-Modalities. That's why they work semantically. That is, the meta-modality distinctions such as close or far sets certain frames of meaning, in this case, that of the conceptual meaning of "distance."

Finally, around the same time, another meta-level model that was created in NLP was the Meta-Program Model. This refers to the perceptual filters, thinking patterns, or point-of-view distinctions that a person uses in sorting for and filtering representations. In Cognitive psychology, meta-programs are most commonly referred to as thinking patterns, frames of mind, perceptual lens, etc. And obviously, they influence what we see and how we experience it.

Actualizing Experiences of Excellence

When high levels meaning are incorporated in certain experiences—they are revealed in best practices, in peak performances, in that which is highest and best in those individuals who push the limits and move to what we call "world class" experiences. In this instance, high quality meaning already exists and is already showing up via someone's neurology. Here we don't have to imagine, create, or invent meaning—we only have to discover it. We only have to model what it is and how it works. And when we articulate it, we can then work with it— refine it and turn it into actionable steps so others can experience it. This describes what *modeling* is.

Modeling Projects that Led to Neuro-Semantics

As I completed my trainings in NLP, Richard Bandler challenged me to do a modeling project. So with the Strategy Model in hand, along with the linguistic model of the Meta-Model, Meta-Programs, and Sub-Modalities, I began my very first modeling project. I wanted to fully understand *resilience* as a human experience of excellence—its structure, strategy, how it worked, and how it could be replicated into the lives of others. To that end I began studying resilience in 1991 and continued until 1994. In 1994 I thought I had completed the project and so presented it in a workshop at the NLP Conference in Denver. What I did not know at the time was that I had missed the multi-level dimensions of resilience.

The realization occurred as I was presenting my current level of conclusions. I first identified the stages of resilience and the realization that resilience is not a simple or single state. It involves a series of states as a person recovers from the emotional roller-coaster of a set-back and then moves through the stages of shock, denial, bargaining, depression, and acceptance (the grief stages of Elizabeth Kubler-Ross). Resilience requires that a person has something to be resilient about—a new vision, a new dream, and the energy within that puts "bounce" back into a person.

Then, as I had done for several years, I used the elicitation question which I had used a hundred times before. To make the workshop experimental and related to real life, I asked for a volunteer. My intention was to demonstrate the natural stages and steps of resilience.

> "Who has been through hell and back? Who has been knocked down, but today you are back, having fully recovered and now you are a living example of resilience?"

But then as the conversation ensued, something new happened. As I was questioning and exploring with the gentleman who had volunteered, at one point I asked him, "How did you know that you were ready to move from this stage to the next one? How were you able to do that?"

His explanation was so simple, I could have easily missed it. But having spent time reading and re-reading Gregory Bateson's *Steps to an Ecology of Mind* and Alfred Korzybski's *Science and Sanity,* I was primed to listen for and detect levels. And that's what I heard when the gentleman spoke:

> "I just knew that I will get through this, it was like I had a higher state, a meta-state about the state I was in, so that I knew this too would pass and I would get through it, and that things would be okay for me."

From that conversation in that workshop experience the Meta-States Model rose in my mind. Within the week that followed, I wrote a forty-page document detailing out Meta-States as a model and sent it off to the NLP Trainers Association as a contribution to the NLP model. Later Wyatt Woodsmall and the Association recognized the Meta-States Model as "the most significant model that complemented the NLP model in 1995." That was my first modeling project. It was not the last.

How Meta-States Re-Modeled NLP
From the modeling of resilience came the Meta-States Model which then took the modeling that we do in Neuro-Semantics to a whole new level. At that time I didn't know that. What I was doing consciously at the time was explicitly mapping out the NLP model with Bob Bodenhamer. We took the models of NLP and by viewing them through the lens of Meta-States, began writing books to present the models as straight forward as we could. What then happened was unexpected and unintended: we re-modeled NLP itself.

We began with the Time-Line patterns, then Sleight of Mouth patterns, then Meta-Programs, and finally Sub-Modalities. And with each book, we found that using the Meta-States Model it kept re-modeling NLP making it more streamlined and simplifying the processes. This allowed us to articulate the meta-level structures that NLP had not been able to do.[3] And eventually this led to the series of books that Bob and I co-authored:

> *Adventures in Time*
> *Mind-Lines: Lines for Changing Minds*
> *Figuring Out People*
> *Sub-Modalities Going Meta*

Finally, we put together the basic textbooks for NLP Practitioner course and Master Practitioner Course (*User's Manual of the Brain, Volumes I and II*). Then as a way to simplify the Meta-States Model, I then began modeling the structure of meaning via one's self-reflexivity and that led to writing, *Frame Games* (now, *Winning the Inner Game,* 2007). And with the Framing Model, that led to a whole series of books and trainings:

> *Games for Mastering Fear*
> *Games Fit and Slim People Play*
> *Games Great Lovers Play*
> *Games Business Experts Play*
> *Games for Accelerated Learning*
> *Games for Prolific Writing, etc.*

The next modeling that developed new Neuro-Semantic models was the modeling of self-actualization. That led to the *Axes of Change Model, the Self-Actualization Axes and Quadrants, the Volcano Hierarchy of Needs* (Matrix-Embedded Pyramid) etc.

Neuro-Semantics and Modeling Projects

After discovering the Meta-States Model, I began using my research skills to look for, discover, and articulate other experiences of excellence. My interest at that time was to identify certain experiences of expertise that I needed for myself, like resilience. In fact, that became one of the criteria I always used with the creation of a new model:

•   Does it work for me?

•   If I applied to myself, could I access the new experience to enrich my own life?

If so, then it would meet the test and I knew that I was really ready to offer it to others. That initiated me into becoming a modeler of positive psychological experiences that, like resilience, would be useful for myself and others. That lead me to model creativity, writing (and also best sellers), women in leadership, sales, wealth creation, coaching, self-actualization, self-actualizing leaders and companies, etc.   And from all of this came the creation of many models which today make up Neuro-Semantics such as the Meta-States Model, the Matrix Model, the Axes of Change model, and the Meta-Coach Training system, etc. Most of these eventually became books or training manuals as well as trainings.

1992-1994	1) Resilience	Resilience and *Meta-States* (2008)
1992-1996	2) Reflexivity	*Meta-States* (2008), *Dragon Slaying* (2000)
1996	3) Sales, Selling	Selling Genius
1995-1996	4) State Management	*Dragon Slaying;* Defusing Hotheads
1996-1997	5) Meaning / Frames	*Mind-Lines* (1997/2005)*; Frame Games* (1999)
1997-1998	6) Women in Leadership	With Dr. Jennifer Hays, Baylor Medical University; Jeff Hays
1997-1999	7) Wealth Creation	*Inside-Out Wealth* (2010)
1997-2003	8) Entrepreneurs	
2000-2001	9) Weight Mgmt. and Fitness	*Games Slim and Fit People Play* (2001)
2000	10) Writing Skills and Best Sellers	*Prolific Writing*
2001	11) Business Leaders	*Games Business Experts Play* (2002)
2001	12) Culture	Cultural Modeling
2001-2009	13) Coaching	*Meta-Coaching Series*
2003-2004	14) Change / Transformation	*Coaching Change* (2003)
2003-2009	15) Self-Actualization	*Unleashed* (2007), *Self-Actualization Psychology* (2008), *Achieving Peak Performance* (2009)
2007-2009	16) Self-Actualization Leadership	*Unleashing Leadership* (2009)
2009-2011	17) Benchmarking	*Benchmarking Intangibles*
2009-2011	18) Meaning	*Neuro-Semantics*

Principles for Modeling

While modeling is an advanced skill in meaning detection and explication, there are some basic principles that govern this competency.[4] What do you need to know to model? What do you need to do? What attitude and orientation do you need to adopt so that you can take an experience and make a model or map of how it works that someone could use to reproduce that experience?

1) Model to a well-formed outcome.

What do you want to model? What experience that someone does with excellence or that could be done with excellence? Model for an outcome. Model for the purpose of finding or creating a model about how a person can do or experience something. What will the model ultimately give you? What outcome do you want to achieve? Do you have a well-formed outcome for your modeling so that you can tell what is relevant and what is not relevant to the model that you want to produce?

What are you seeking to model—a person, an experience, or a product? Wyatt Woodsmall distinguishes these kinds of modeling. You can model a person— his or her attitude, spirit, and higher states. You can model what a person creates, the products that result from the person.

2) Begin your modeling by mimicking.

Spend time observing someone and see if you can mimic them. Can you reproduce their actions, voice, and external responses? Effectively modeling often requires that you develop your sensory acuity and flexibility to sense and reproduce what you sense (what you see, hear, feel, move, etc.). As you *identify* with the person and adopt more and more of his or her responses, what thoughts and emotions emerge, what has to be true to operate this way?

Begin also by extensively researching what has already been discovered about the experience or skill. Who else has studied this? Written on it? Who are the key thinkers as indicated by the literature of the field?

Model from the right states. If it is observing— their intense curiosity, know-nothing state, detective exploration, etc. If it is studying and research, then focus and fascination. If it is mimicking someone, then in a state of respect, rapport, empathy.

3) Detect the hidden patterns that are enabling the experience or skill.

Beyond what you can see and hear externally, what are the hidden patterns that are governing the experience? What patterns of thinking, believing, understanding, deciding, etc. are within the experience? Explore with a thousand question about what the person is doing inside, mentally, emotionally, volitionally, etc. to create the experience. What is the structuring and sequencing of the variables that create the experience? In exploration of unconscious competence, ask lots of questions to tease out the pattern behind the experience.

4) Detect the hidden layers within the experience.

The patterning may be a pattern of the syntax of how the layers of mind are sequenced. What are the beliefs that support the first level belief? What are the higher intentions above and beyond the first level intentions? As you identify frames within the person's mind, and as you hold that frame, what are the frames that transcend that frame?

5) Identify the variables and processes.

After identifying the variables and elements in an experience, list them and then reduce them as you search for the fewest variables that are necessary to create the experience. The fewest distinctions necessary is called modeling "elegance." What are the processes? How many steps are involved? Are there more than one stage? If so, how many stages and phases in the process?

What are the key variables that you will be using and sequencing? NLP begins with the representational systems, the TOTE model for sequencing, the Meta-Model for questioning and de-nominalizing vague terminology. What is incidental or even accidental to the strategy?

6) Solidify your tentative guess about the structure.

Do you know when to begin, where to begin? Do you know when to end? Your model will need the beginning place of the experience and the ending when it has completed its sequence. Do you know how to punctuate the starting and stopping places?

Formulate the structure with the S-R model (Stimulus- Response). This will give you a basic strategy. Model by eliciting and describing the strategy. This is where modeling begins. First model one person's strategy, then another, then several more strategies for the same experience. When you have several, then step back to identify what is sufficient and necessary about the strategy; afterwards you can then work on streamlining the strategy and adding other resources to create a model of the experience.

7) Look for the transcending of levels and systemic processes.

Within human experiences, there is self-reflexive awareness that creates the layers of frames. What logical levels are within the experience? In terms of the mind-body-emotion system, what are the systemic processes that you are dealing with? Where are the boundaries, forces, leverage points, feed back, feed forward lops, emergence, etc. in the system? How do the levels interface with each other to create new emergent properties?

With systemic structures, the structure is dynamic rather than static. It moves, it changes, it evolves. No matter how dynamic an experience, we can model its structure. This is true of tornados, the way a baseball player hits and runs, how a mathematician thinks, how we depress, panic, and traumatize ourselves.

Neuro-Semantic Learnings for a Neuro-Semanticist

Modeling lies at the heart of Neuro-Semantics as it does for NLP and as it did for the first Human Potential Movement. This refers to finding best practices or examples of excellence and exploring the structure of meaning that facilitates and enables that performance.

1) What would you love to model? If you open your eyes and ears, what exemplars of excellence do you find in your world that you would like to know how it works and how you can adopt it for yourself? As you identify the experience that is humanly possible, what meaning (understanding, believing, deciding, etc.) is that experience actualizing or manifesting? How is that happening?

2) Take the modeling principles listed in this chapter and begin exploring how you can use these principles to model some best practice that you want for yourself.

End of Chapter Notes

1. You can find a full description of the strategy model in the book, *NLP: Volume I* by Robert Dilts. I modeled *NLP Going Meta* after that book.

2. See *Sub-Modalities Going Meta* (1999/ 2005) for a full history of the story of sub-modalities and especially on how they work semantically.

3. There were others in NLP who did explore meta-levels in NLP: Robert Dilts, Conneirae Andreas.

4. For the Neuro-Semantic books on modeling, see the following:
    The Matrix Model (2003)
    NLP Going Meta (2005)
    Advanced Neuro-Semantic Model Training Manual
    Cultural Model – Training Manual
    Advanced Flexibility – Training Manual
    Benchmarking Intangibles (2011)

Chapter 18

BECOMING A SKILLED

NEURO-SEMANTICIST

Me— a Neuro-Semanticist?

If Neuro-Semantics is about actualizing your highest meanings into your best performances, then becoming a skillfully competent Neuro-Semanticist, presupposes developing several semantic skills. What's required for this? What knowledge content, insights, skills, ethics, and so on are prerequisites for this? Having been introduced to these skills in the previous chapters, here is a summary. This summary answers the question, "What are the semantic competencies I need in order to think and effectively influence people as a Neuro-Semanticist?"

Insights for Neuro-Semanticists
Throughout the pages of this book numerous insights have been offered. To highlight those that are especially important for a Neuro-Semanticist, I have created the following list:
• Meaning doesn't exist —at least it does not exist "out there."
• Meaning is an inside-out job— you create it.
• Meaning is created neuro-linguistically— in your neurology using the symbolism of language to stand for something other than itself.
• You cannot *not* create meaning— You are a meaning-maker.

- Humans have no instinct, except the "instinct" of creating meaning (learning, making sense of things).
- The meaning your create is the instinct you live.
- You semantically load and unload events, experiences, people, words.
- In a semantic reaction, a meaning controls you and you just react.
- In a semantic response, you choose and control your meanings.
- The quality of your meanings is the quality of your life.
- You are never stuck with any particular meaning—you can always deframe and reframe a meaning.
- The meaning you set is the frame you live.
- It takes a lot of self-esteem, value, and meaning to get the ego out of the way—and to be humble.
- You have to be meta-mindful to fully self-actualize your potentials.
- The frames you create compose the reality you live.
- There's plasticity to meaning; meanings are fluid, that's why you can transform them with ease and grace.
- The meaning you create is the emotion you feel.
- Emotions are the somatizing of your meanings.
- By your conversations you communicate your meanings.

The Basic Set of Neuro-Semantic Competencies
Here now is a set of competencies that will give you tremendous ability as a meaning-maker in working with meanings.

1) Detecting Meaning Competency
First is the ability to *recognize* a frame as a person's interpretative scheme. This means the ability to recognize that there are different kinds, levels, and dimensions of meanings and to distinguish specific differences within each of these categories. The kinds of meanings range from different representations, labels, classifications, metaphors, etc. (chapter 3). The different levels range from the un-speakable level to the self-reflexive levels created by meta-stating (chapter 4). This skill also involves recognizing meanings as coded in emotions, habits, and beliefs (chapter 5).

It all begins here. If you can't recognize meaning as it shows up in yourself, others, and the world, it will control you. At the heart of this skill is the ability to recognize that whatever a person says that something is, it is not. Those are just the words that person attributes to the thing.

2) Exploring Meanings Competency

From detection arises the skill of exploring meanings—yours, others, the cultures you live in, etc. This skill centers in asking meta-questions and begins when you embrace another person's semantic reality. Do this even if that semantic reality is classified as a "problem" or a "complaint" (chapter 7). Curiously explore how it works and what it generates without any evaluation about the person or the meaning. This skill operates best in you when it comes from the premise: If there's a problem, the frame is the problem, not the person. The person is never the problem; the frame is always the problem.

3) Creating (Constructing, Inventing) Meaning Competency

Now given the different kinds, levels, and dimensions of meaning, you can develop your skill in creating meanings. This skill entails being able to create coherence, order, and structure out of experiences (chapters 2-5), frames and reframes (chapter 14), and develop your narrative competence (chapter 15). As this skill develops so will your speed and flexibility in constructing meaning increases thereby enabling you to do it in real time at those moments when you need to generate new meanings (chapter 7).

4) Climbing the Ladder of Meaning Competency

With the ability to detect, explore, and hold meanings, you can now climb the ladder of meaning and explore a whole matrix of meaning. This skill makes your self-reflexive consciousness useful and practical as you move up, level after level, to explore and map out how the semantic landscape in yourself, in another, or in a cultural context works.

5) Quality Controlling Meanings Competency

This refers to the skill of stepping aside from a meaning or frame to check its ecology, evaluate it systemically, and run a checklist on cognitive distortions. And when you can do that, you'll also be able to clean up cognitive distortions which you may find that are interfering with full humanness (chapter 6).

6) Holding a Frame of Meaning Competency

This semantic skill refers to being able to hold a frame stable for yourself or another person in a conversation so that the person can then respond or reflect about it. Doing this enables you to reveal or discover the next level frame. To do this, accept whatever is offered you and repeat it back for the person's acknowledgment and confirmation (chapter 12). Typically this requires slowing yourself down and not being semantically reactive. As you *go with* someone's meanings, it doesn't mean you are condoning them, just seeking to understand them.

7) Broadening Meaning Competency

Expanding what else a particular meaning, understanding, idea, etc. could mean is the semantic skill by which you can make a meaning richer, fuller, more robust, more useful, and so on. This skill involves the ability to semantically load a meaning (chapter 6). In involves the ability to expand the number of meanings that you give to an event, person, word, etc. and thus your flexibility in generating more and more meanings (chapter 7).

8) Suspending (Releasing) Meaning Competency

This important semantic skill refers to the ability to invalidate an old meaning by suspending it, deframing it, releasing it, negating it, and so on (chapter 13). Without the ability to suspend or release a meaning, you are the subject of the meaning, rather than the meaning being subject to you. This skill includes the ability to question a frame in such a way as to loosen the frames that hold limiting meanings. You can unload the semantic meanings that have overloaded something.

9) Monitoring Meanings Competency

Monitoring a frame or meaning refers to observing and tracking how a meaning works out over time in your life or the life of another. Meanings are fluid. They evolve, change, and transmute. How does a meaning change over course of an experience or even a conversation? Meaning doesn't hold still. Like a living, breathing, evolving entity, it can morph to become a very different content. At an advanced level, this skill involves using your self-reflexive awareness to follow a meaning through a matrix of frames (tracking through the Matrix Model).

10) Scaling Meaning Competency

Because all meaning is not the same, you can learn to distinguish it in its numerous forms. The ability to scale meaning involves measuring meaning (its kind, level, intensity, quality, etc.). This skill can entail using a scale to recognize the levels of a meaning (chapter 6). It may involve recognizing different kinds of meanings (chapter 4). It may involve recognizing degrees of conditionality of meanings (chapter 7).

11) Sacrilizing Competency

Sacrilizing refers to the ability to see a person, event, word, etc. "under the aspect of eternity." That is, to see its ultimate value and importance and to thereby appreciate it, to see it as valuable in and of itself apart from its instrumental value. This skill enables you to see things with a fresh appreciation (chapter 6). You can also now semantically load something with rich and robust meanings so that it offers a rejuvenating source of inspiration to yourself and others (chapters 3, 6, and 11).

12) Holding Meaningful Conversations Competency

To speak, to transmit thoughts, to exchange ideas, etc. engages in the heart of meaning-making— conversation. What makes this magical is that in conversation you communicate the meanings of your mind to the minds of others. Your information can literally *in-form* others—forming them in accordance with the meanings that you offer. Your words and non-verbals can not only frame, but also deframe, reframe, and outframe (chapter 16).

Summary of Patterns

Numerous patterns were presented throughout the text, here is a list of the formal patterns that gives you tremendous power within you meaning-making and patterns for Coaching Conversations to facilitate the self-actualizing of potentials in others.

Chapter 6	Cleaning up Cognitive Distortions Pattern
Chapter 9	Self-Actualization Assessment Scale
Chapter 10	Meaningful to the Core Pattern
Chapter 11	Peak Experience Detection and Utilization Pattern
	Making it Meaningful Pattern
	Meaning Enrichment Pattern
	Developing your Meta-Needs Pattern
	Expanding Meta-Programs Pattern
Chapter 12	Into the Construct Pattern
	Coaching for Matrix Detection Pattern
	Opening up a Belief System Pattern
Chapter 13	The Art of Deframing
	Meta-Model Questioning Pattern
	Releasing Semantic Reactivity Pattern
	Movie Rewind Pattern
	Drop Down Through Pattern

Neuro-Semantic Learnings for a Neuro-Semanticist

Now you know what *it* is. And now the adventure can begin in earnest as you take these insights, these skills, and these patterns into the real world of your home, friendships, hobbies, and business. Now you can strategically work and play to bring out your highest values and visions and make them real in your best performances.

Appendix A

NEURO-SEMANTIC MODELS

1) Meta-States Model
Chapter 1, 3, 4, 5, 17

2) Frame Games Model
Chapter 1, 4 (p. 63), 17

3) The Matrix Model
Chapter 4

4) Meaning–Performance Axes
Chapter 5, 17

5) Self-Actualization Quadrants
Chapter 5, 17

6) Matrix-Embedded Pyramid
In *Self-Actualization Psychology* and *Unleashed*

7) Axes of Change Model
Chapter 1

8) The Crucible Model
Chapter 1

9) Mind-Lines Model
Chapter 14

10) The Meta-Dimensions Model
Appendix C

Appendix B

NEURO-SEMANTIC BOOKS

The following are basic books about Neuro-Semantics.

Meta-States: Managing the Higher Levels of Your Self-Reflective Consciousness.
> This was the first Neuro-Semantic book. It details the discovery of Meta-States in the context of the resilience modeling project.

Mind-Lines: Lines for Changing Minds.
> The first book that applied the Meta-States Model to the linguistic distinctions in NLP for creating influence in language, the "sleight of mouth" patterns.

Secrets of Personal Mastery.
> The title of this book was originally to be "Secrets of Personal Genius" to correspond to the training, Accessing Personal Genius (APG). It presents the basic Meta-States model and patterns presented in APG.

Frame Games, now titled, *Winning the Inner Game.*
> A user-friendly version of Meta-States using "games" for states and "frames" for the meta or higher levels. From this came a whole series of books and training manuals: *Games for Mastering Fear, Games Fit and Slim People Play, Games Great Lovers Play, Games Business Experts Play,* etc.

The Matrix Model.
> From Frame Games arose the Matrix Model as a systems model for all of the patterns in NLP and Neuro-Semantics. The Matrix refers to the collection of process and content frames that make up our "model of the world" and which govern our sense of reality and the source of our responses.

The NLP Re-Modeled Books.
>   This series of books arose quite by accident as Bob Bodenhamer and I began applying the Meta-States Model to the basic models of NLP. *Mind-Lines* was first, then *Adventures in Time, Figuring Out People* (on Meta-Programs), *Sub-Modalities Going Meta, User's Manual of the Brain, Volumes I and II.*

The Meta-Coaching Series.
>   This series of books began in 2003 to detail out the Neuro-Semantic approach to Coaching.

Ordering Books
Most of the books can be obtained through Amazon.com. Otherwise you can order them through the following publishers. For the catalogue, go to www.neurosemantics.com.

NSP: Neuro-Semantic Publications
P.O. Box 8
Clifton, Colorado, USA 81520–0008
(970) 523-7877
Email: meta@acsol.net

CHP: Crown House Publishing
6 Trowbridge Drive, Suite 5
Bethel, CT. 06801
Phone: 203-778-1300
email: mtracten@chpus.com

Appendix C

The Meta-Dimensions

Towards a Unified Field Theory

When I began exploring meta-states and meta-levels, I began with the four levels in Robert Dilts model (i.e., beliefs, values, identity, spiritual)[1] and within a very short time, I identified 15 or more levels. Given that these levels were already there, that part was easy. The problem at that point was trying to figure out a way to communicate the multiple distinctions of the levels and *how they relate to each other*. That was harder.[2]

Later, when I developed the *Mind-Lines Model*, I took the 14 patterns of NLP (called "the sleight of mouth" patterns) and expanded them to 20 and using the Meta-States model, I set them up as meta-levels for outframing. At the time, I thought that was pretty exhaustive. What I later discovered was that it was just exhaustive of my mind at that moment in time![3]

Later with the development of Meta-Coaching, I put the meta-level distinctions into the form of *meta-questions* and expanded it to 26. Then I found a couple more, then Denis Bridoux suggested another couple. Now we were up to 30, then there were 38. As you will see later, the list has now extended to over 100 meta-level distinctions. That obviously goes beyond the $7^{+/-2}$ distinctions that we normally can handle.

What's a meta-person to do? What's a Meta-Coach to do? What's a Neuro-Semanticist to do?[4] These questions initiated yet another new search.
>"If I collected and categorized all of the meta-levels and sort them out into a new classification form, what form would that take? How are the levels related? What is the relationship between the scores and scores of words and terms that refer to various meta-phenomena? Are there any layer level classifications, domains, or dimensions above the specific levels?"

It was this exploration that got me interested in understanding and mapping out the dimension of the mind's meta-levels. It was as if I had been doing this for years yet without having done it explicitly. The time had now come to do that.

Metaphors of Meta Land

As I did, I revisited the various metaphors that we already have and that we've developed to model this area. So what are the *metaphors* that seek to describe *the phenomena* at the meta-levels? Dilts began by using a *hierarchical pyramid*. But that metaphor is far too static, staid, and un-dynamic and un-systemic to describe the systemic interactive nature of the meta-levels. So I first used the *height* metaphor of reflexivity by which we reflexively apply back to ourselves one layer upon another layer of thoughts-and-feelings. That led to the frame games metaphor of *frames embedded in frames* and a framework of personality. Yet because this was still mostly static, I was not satisfied with that metaphor.

Next came the *diamond* metaphor. Here playing off of the idea that each meta-level is but another *facet* of the same subjective experience only from a different view, the image of the *diamond of consciousness* provided a more three-dimensional and dynamic approach. With the *matrix metaphor*, an even more energetic, dynamic, and systemic feel was brought to the meta-levels. That helped considerably. We can now draw pictures and diagrams of an emerging and evolving system of these meta-levels.

Within all of the Neuro-Semantic metaphors is the *spiraling and circling metaphor* of a eddy of water or *tornado* that moves both upward with more of the same and then downward. This metaphor allows the system dynamics of feed back and feed forward loops to be portrayed with much more clarity. It also allows us an image of the ongoing evolution of the system with each layering. Next, in the development of some of the Self-Actualization models, the *onion metaphor* emerged. This metaphor enables us to convey that the layering is made out of the same living stuff at each level and that by unpeeling an onion of meaning we can get to the core of things — the original thoughts-and-feelings that created the reflexive system of meaning.

With all of these metaphors, we have been getting closer to understanding the landscape of the meta-levels of our minds. The multiple metaphors enable us to think and talk about the world of reflexivity layering thoughts-and-feelings that build up the matrix of our meaning frames and giving us multiple perspectives or facets for entering the system so that we can get to the heart of things.

Since discovering the *reflexivity process* deep inside the basic Meta-States Model, it has been clear that there's no hierarchy to the meta-levels. It is more of *a holoarchy*—another metaphor. A holoarchy is a dynamic structure of wholes in parts in such a way that every whole is part of a yet higher whole. As a whole, it is a embedded within layers of wholes. This explains why the question, "Which is the highest level?" is a pseudo-question an irrelevant one.

When it comes to the meta-levels, no level is higher than another level. That's because we can *reflexively* always step back and outframe whatever we have experienced with yet another. Do you think *identity* is higher than *belief*. If so, can you have a *belief* about your *identity*? Can you *value* your *spirit*? It is our self-reflexive consciousness which prevents one level from being higher than another level. It does this because we can always reflect back on any level with another. This infinite regress of our self-reflexive conscious means we can always meta-state any level with any other level.

Dimensions of Meta-Levels

So while no one single *level* is higher than another, what about the existence of different *dimensions* of meta-phenomena? Could there be areas of meta-levels by which we can describe the landscape of various dimensions within the landscape of *meta*?

Suppose that there are some basic *dimensions* that can help us map out the territory of *meta*. What would be the difference between a level or a dimension?

> A *level* is any thought or feeling, any distinction that we can layer upon other thoughts and feelings. That creates another *level*. And there are now over 100 of these levels. Sometimes we call them "logical levels" and sometimes we refer to them as our psycho-logics, that is, our psycho-logical levels.

> A *dimension,* on the other hand, describes not just levels, but many levels. It is an area of levels wherein the meta-levels within operate at a certain stage of development. So within the area there will be a whole set of new distinctions with new dynamics and processes.

So while there's no hierarchy to the levels, they are totally fluid, there is a hierarchy of development of the dimensions.

The hierarchical nature of the *meta-dimensions* arises from the cognitive or mental development we all go through. Piaget was the first pioneer in Developmental Psychology that began mapping out the *stages* of cognitive development speaking about representational constancy, to concrete thinking, pre-formal operations, formal operations, etc. Erickson pioneered the psycho-social stages and Fowler the faith or moral stages.

Regarding terminology, I have chosen to call these *Meta-Dimensions* rather than *Meta-Domains* although my first preference would be the term "domain." The problem, however, is that I have used the phrase *meta-domain* for some ten years to refer to some of *the areas of study* in NLP. When I entered the field, there were two meta-domains: the Meta-Model of Language in Therapy and Meta-Programs. I introduced Meta-States to the field in 1994 as the third meta-domain. Later I discovered that sub-modalities were not *lower* or *sub* at all, but itself another meta-domain. That gives us four "meta-domains." Although as you will notice, the Meta-Model and the Meta-Modalities of the cinematic features (the sub-modalities) fits into the Representational dimension, Meta-Programs into the Gestalt dimension, Meta-States in the Meta-States dimension and the Conceptual dimension.[5]

The dimensions gives a way of navigating the landscape of the meta-levels:

- Representation dimension
- Meta-State dimension
- Gestalt dimension
- Conceptual dimension

I: The Representational Dimension

We begin with the area of representational reality because before the meta processes occur, the structure and content of our consciousness consists simply of representations. We bring the outside world that we detect through our senses and sense receptors (eyes, ears, nose, mouth, skin, inner ear, etc.) and even before awareness or words, the various parts of our cortex are processing the data from the world "out there." Our visual cortex, auditory cortex, motor cortex, etc. actively work as our cognitive unconscious giving us our first access to external reality, building up our neurological maps. As we become conscious of the content of sights, sounds, and sensations in our "stream of consciousness" we have the experience of seeing, hearing, sensing, smelling, tasting, etc. a world on the inside of our mind. It is as if we have a screen on the theater of our mind and can *present to ourselves again* (re-presentation) what we have seen and heard before. (see *MovieMind*, 2002).

Regarding this dimension, psychologists have long tried to bring order to it. Yet it was the genius of NLP that named the *internal representations* as the "languages of the mind" and put them together as a communication model. Bateson noted this is his Preface to *The Structure of Magic* (1975) complimenting Bandler and Grinder on this breakthrough. They had found something to be the basis of consciousness which could lead to practical processes for running one's own brain and managing consciousness and its states. They had found our internal mapping of the senses.[6]

In the Representational Dimension we 'think" by using our representational systems to create snapshots and movies in our mind, and when we become elegant, we can put in a sound track with the tones, volumes, and other auditory qualities that facilitate our understanding. Then we can step in or out of the movie at choice depending on what we want to do with our inner movies. In this dimension also includes the meta-representational system of language —linguistics, mathematics, and other abstract representations.

When we step back from our movies, we are able to notice the *modes of thought* (i.e., the modalities) that make up the movies as well as the meta-modality (i.e., the sub-modalities) distinctions in each system. This enables us to take charge of *editing* our movies. Here we are at a meta-level, the *editorial level* of choosing how to encode or program the movie. So even at this first level, the Representational dimension contains meta-processes. Yet because everything is focused on the Movie, the content of the Movie, and we are basically still mostly in reference to the Movie in terms of the outside world, we are mostly working with *the basic sensory and lingusitic representation*s.

Relating this to the Matrix Model, the grounding matrix of State occurs here in the Representational dimension. In the Mind-Lines Model, the framing, reframing, and deframing patterns occur here.

II: The Meta-State Dimension
Even though self-reflexivity operates in the area of representations, when we shift our focus from *the content* of our thinking and responding to *our*

responding itself, we move fully into the Meta-State dimension. In this dimension we are more concerned about our thinking and feeling. If we felt fear about something "out there" in the world, now we might feel *embarrassed* about our fear, *angry* at our fear, *guilty* for fearing, *proud* of the fear, *afraid* of our fear, or a hundred other responses.

Our consciousness at this first simple level of meta-stating is very fluid as it is at the Representational dimension. Thoughts, feelings, memories, and imaginations come and go like a "stream of consciousness" (William James' descriptive phrase). Here also, we experience a lot of emotion. Untrue to what some in NLP have asserted, "going meta" is *not* the same as the so-called phenomenon of "dissociation." As the example in the previous paragraph—being embarrassed about our fear or angering at our fear does not create numbness, but more emotions so that we become more emotional, not less.

The Meta-State dimension is the domain of accessing and applying other thoughts, feelings, and even physiology (physiological responses as in how we use our body, breath, move, gesture, etc.) to our previous thoughts. Structurally, this creates layers and layers of texture upon our primary states. Now our *confidence*, for example, can be textured with respect, humor, lightness, awareness of fallibility, contextual awareness, etc. Equally, it could be textured with superiority, demandingness, and irritation of others who are not as competent. The *texture* of our experiences refer to the meta-states that we've accessed and applied. They speak about the quality and property of the state. So in this, *calm anger* differs significantly from *intolerant anger.* *Thoughtful fear* is so different from *feared fear.*[7]

In the Meta-State dimension, when we bring thoughts-and-feelings of *confirmation* to other thoughts or feelings, we create *a first-level "belief."* This was what I discovered in Neuro-Semantics more than a decade ago about the structure of a "belief." Today in Neuro-Semantics we recognize a *belief* as a dynamic meta-state, one that emerges when we meta-state our thoughts with *confirmation.* Accessing the sense and feeling of a "confirmation" — that something *is,* that something is true, that that's the way the world is, that something is real — sets a frame over the thought so that we see it, perceive it, feel it, and respond to it as "real." Doing this creates a *belief.*

As such, this distinguishes *a mere thought* from *a belief.* We can *think* all kinds of things. We can think, imagine, represent, and encode in multiple ways all kinds of things that we don't believe. A belief, in contrast to a thought, engages and commits us. When we believe something, we strongly feel that something is so. We feel a sense of *conviction* about it as much more of our neurology is involved in a belief.

First-level beliefs operate much more dynamically and powerfully than just thoughts. Thoughts certainly send *messages* to our body, but beliefs send *commands* to our nervous system. As such beliefs can have tremendous effects upon our health, well-being, and functioning. That's precisely why limiting and morbid beliefs can be so damaging and create severe interferences. Beliefs operate as self-organizing frames that create self-fulfilling prophecies.[8]

In the Matrix Model, the central two process matrices of Meaning and Intention occur in the Meta-State dimension. This describes the levels of the meaning-making processes within us. In the Mind-Lines Model, all of the outframing patterns occur here.

III: The Gestalt Dimension

While first-level beliefs are dynamic and emotional, they introduce a new distinction about the meta-levels. The distinction is that in meta-stating *confirmation,* the thought becomes something more than just a higher level state, it becomes *a gestalt state.* This means it operates as a *whole* so that the confirmed-thought as a belief commands and governs the nervous system. It also operates as a form of consciousness that we now "hold" in mind. Consciousness now ceases to be fluid. It settles down so that we experience it as more staid and solid. Because the "belief" as a gestalt state now *holds* a particular content in our mind— it is our "meaning" ("meaning" means "to hold in mind").

In the Gestalt dimension when we have these very complex states operating as a whole, they feel and function in a way similar to a primary state. So self-esteem, proactivity, responsibility, uninsultability, etc. operate as if they were one thing, and not layers upon layers of complex understandings. As they have been gestalted, the variables coalesce together into a whole. Now "the sum of all the parts is greater than all those parts."

To meta-state several layers in such a way that the experience gestalts requires a certain elegance in the meta-stating. It requires the ability to hold constant the nugget of the experience while layering it with various qualities and doing so until it coalesces for the person and is felt as a *whole,* as one singular state. When that happens, it becomes not only a belief, but a belief-system, a dynamic hologram. So if you are meta-stating the experience of a "set-back in life" and wanting the meta-state of *resilience* to emerge from the process, you hold constant the set-back experience in order to ground resilience to the context. Then you layer ideas that grow into beliefs about acceptance of life, the openness to just witnessing, the self-efficacy of trusting oneself and one's resources, the importance of actualizing one's dreams and passions, the importance of persistence, etc.[9]

Every gestalt state is made up of beliefs within belief systems. And what is a belief system? A *belief system is a system of beliefs embedded inside of other beliefs so that there's a whole system of inter-connected beliefs supporting a single idea.* Realizing this, ten years ago I created the Meta-State pattern, *Opening Up a Belief System* (pp. 204-206). A belief system, represents a higher level of meta-stating, involves the creation of multiple *gestalt states.* And as such, it is a higher dimension of meta-levels than all of the first level of meta-levels.

The gestalting process that takes one or more variables and enables them to coalesce into a singular whole. *This is the very process by which our meta-states become meta-programs.* As a perceptual filter, the Meta-Programs model identifies those conceptual, emotional, conative, and semantic *lens* that we use to look at and perceive the world. As such, meta-programs governs what we select to notice. So where do these meta-programs come from? For the most part we *meta-state* them into existence.[10]

For example, consider the meta-programs on the continuum from specific to general. We speak of the first as the mindset and thinking of *detailing* and the other as *global thinking.* This refers to the level of specificity / abstraction that we prefer and whether we prefer to use inductive or deductive reasoning as we draw conclusions. The *detail* perceiver sees the trees rather than the forest whereas the *global* perceiver sees the forest rather than the trees. So one brings a detailing state to the inner movies and zooms in; the other brings a global state and zooms out to get a larger picture. As each then meta-states such with value, they become more committed to that way of perceiving and thinking. As they meta-state with identifying, they begin identifying themselves as that kind of person. When all of these coalesces, it creates the gestalt of operating as a perceptual filter.

IV: The Conceptual Dimension

Above and beyond the Gestalt dimension is the area where beliefs and belief-systems become so much "the way it is," that we experience them without much emotion at all. Emotion, which becomes much less pronounced in the Gestalt dimension, becomes almost entirely absent in the Conceptual dimension. If beliefs grow up to become belief-systems, what do belief-systems grow up to become? The answer is Conceptual or Semantic systems.

Sometimes when I work with a person, I will ask about something important and then listen to how the person expresses the belief. After pacing their experience, I will comment, "So you believe that?" I do so to test the strength of conviction in the belief. I want to know the energy intensity of the belief. Typically, the person will go, "Yes, definitely!" But not always. Sometimes the person will go, "No. I don't believe it, I *know* it."

For the longest time I didn't know what to think of that. My first thought was, "Of course, it's a belief. Everything is a belief. It's beliefs all the way up. The person is just not wanting to call it a belief because it feels more than a belief." But now I think that the phrase, *"I know it"* indicates something else, and something different.

If a belief is a command to the nervous system, and a belief-system is a whole gestalt structure that commands even more neurology, governing our emotions and skills and perceptions, then when we graduate from a *belief* to a *concept*—we move up to a yet higher area where we experience our thoughts as *the very fabric of reality*— as the way it is, as that which is just unquestionable. You know we are getting to the highest levels of a person's mapping or your own because of the use of more "end-of-the-map" kind of words and language: "It's *just* this." "It's *only* X." "There's nothing else." "That's it."

Actually, this has been inside of *the Meta-Yes pattern* for belief change for years, but I had never made it explicit until now. We typically begin with the *emotional Yes* and repeat that until it eventually settles down to a more *matter-of-fact Yes.* We then encourage that repetition until you get the neurological feeling in your body of, *"Of Course!"* Actually, this *of-course* feeling is the strongest experience of all. "Of course, that's just the way it is." When you get to this place, your idea is not only believed, strongly believed, gestalted as a whole, it is now assumed and is part of the very *fabric of reality* in your mind-body system. It has become framework. It is your assumptive reality that isn't open for discussion.

What happens when you meet someone who says something at this level that conflicts with yours? We're talking about something far above a counter-belief that you have. We're talking above a gestalted meta-state like resilience or proactivity. We're talking about someone who says something against your *model of the world,* your *conceptual reality,* your *semantic understandings of life.*

At this level and in this dimension, disagreement is expressed in the smile of contempt and the laugh of non-sense. Suppose someone asserts that the human race evolved on Mars and migrated to this Planet 100,000 years ago and that we are all actually Maritans? If someone said that to you with a straight face, how would you respond? Would you feel a strong urge to argue against it as a belief? Would you feel any compulsion to try to set the person straight? Wouldn't you rather just smile to them and then inside laugh it off as ridiculous? By *the laugh* of contempt, we laugh something off that we consider so stupid and non-sensical that it is not even worth our time or trouble to address.

Things at the Conceptual dimension are mapped as so much "the way it is," as what's real and unquestionable that while we don't have much *emotion* as such about it, the feeling we have is extremely robust and strong. *It just feels right and obvious and without question.* Get an idea to that level, to the area of Concepts, and it commands even more neurology.

I think this explains the Haitian voodoo deaths. Those who *believe* in the hexing of the dolls do so not only as a singular belief, but as a belief-system. And more, it is not only a gestalted reality for them, it is their Model of the World, their Semantic Reality, their assumptive reality. Conceptually, it makes sense to them as just the way things are. So when they are cursed by a voodoo hex, there's just no question. Somewhere and somehow in their neurology, the message is sent as an inevitable command—die. And so they do. Non-believers do not. Heathens do not. And when autopsies are conducted, the doctors cannot find any natural cause of death. We sometimes call this the placebo effect— the self-fulfilling prophecy of a strongly held belief.

In the Meta-Programs model, the higher or semantic meta-programs are in the Conceptual dimension. Here Self, Responsibility, Morality, Time, etc. are concepts that we develop and map. We then use them to navigate our fabric of reality.

In the Matrix Model, the five content matrices (self, power, others, time, and world) are in the Conceptual dimension. These are content maps about specific concepts that are so close to us that philosophers like Emanual Kant assumed that they were *a priori,* prior to our birth and built into our consciousness.

In the Mind-Lines Model, the Time framing patterns (preframing and post-framing) occur here in the Conceptual dimension.

Distinguishing the Dimensions

As we move from one meta-dimension to the next, there's development, richer complexity, and different mechanisms that operate in each.

At the Representational dimension, we call forth sights and sounds for our internal Movie. Within the Movie there may be words. We may also have self-talk about the movie.

> When I think about my job, I see the office building, then I start hearing my boss and some of the people I work with. It's like I'm there.

At the dimension of belief, we begin to assert things that may be difficult to see as a movie. Mental things now become more abstract. Language begins to predominate in the way we encode our beliefs.

> I believe I'm a good person.
> I believe in telling the truth.
> I believe I can learn to become an excellent learner and a life-long learner.
> I believe I can make a difference.

At the Gestalt dimension, we create multiple beliefs and link them together as a supporting system. Here there can be layers upon layers of thoughts and feelings, states that have coalesced into a singular state or experience.

I believe I'm a resilient person who has the ego-strength to look at reality without falling apart and taping into my personal resources for coping and mastering, I believe I have the self-efficacy for bouncing back from any set-back.

I believe in being uninsultable in the face of criticism and rejection because it's not about me as a person, that's settled, I'm already a Somebody and unconditionally so and I'm open to feedback, nothing to fear in that.

At the Conceptual dimension the energy and emotion of our beliefs fade into the background resulting in a more matter-of-fact feel and sense of reality. Here we use our intellectual understandings to map reality and to orient ourselves within what we have mapped.

I know the sun will rise tomorrow, that the planet dependably spins around the sun.

I know that I'm mortal and that I will die.

When you read the early NLP literature about beliefs and belief change, Richard Bandler made no distinction between these levels. For example, when he proposed changing beliefs with sub-modalities he used the following as an example of a belief, "Think of a strong belief like 'I believe the sun will rise tomorrow.'"

Yet today we know that such is not an example of a strong belief. It is an *understanding.* It is conceptual knowledge. We *know* that, we don't believe it. After all, what would be the opposite if you didn't believe it? This is *knowledge content* about the everyday life on this planet, namely, the sun rises. It is not a belief about what you can, or cannot, do or what does, or does not, exist. So as an *understanding* or fact of *knowledge,* "I believe the sun will rise tomorrow" is an inadequate comparison. So using that to try to change a limiting or weak belief using the coding devise of the cinematic features of your representations doesn't work.[11]

Summary

Within the realm of *meta,* we have many, many, many *levels.* We have a great many phenomena that are called by a great many terms. This area is sometimes called "logical levels," yet Korzybski, who first described neuro-linguistic and neuro-semantic reality, described them as our psycho-logics, our psycho-logical levels.

These *levels* we layer one upon another as we think, feel, and live inside a neurology that feeds information in and energy out of our mind-body system. These levels also uniquely describe human experience itself. And that's what makes them so important, so crucial, so central to modeling expertise and facilitating self-actualization.

Via these levels, we combine, merge, and synergize all kinds of experiences, from our highest and best states to our lowest and worst states. So what the Meta-States model began mapping out about the phenomena that occur in the landscape of our higher psycho-logics, we have in Neuro-Semantics been mapping out further and further.

With the creation of the *meta-questions*, we began learning to dance around and peak into the jewel of human experience. The meta-questions brought into our awareness more and more of the *diamond of consciousness* and enables us to explore it from many facets. Today we have over 100 and the number keeps growing. Yet how can you track 26 let alone 100-plus?

The answer is the **Meta-Dimensions.** In the land of meta, in the space or landscape of the meta-phenomena, there are dimensions or domains. It is there that the *levels* occur. And within the four *Meta-Dimensions* we have every model, every pattern, and every variable that we work within in Neuro-Semantic NLP.

Each of these *dimensions* describes a different kind of territory or landscape of our mind-body-emotion system. There are different *levels* in each, different mechanisms, different focus, kinds of thoughts, kinds of emotions, neurology, language, and challenges. There are also different processes for deframing constructions and installing new meaning creations. So while there is no hierarchy to the *levels* themselves, there is a hierarchy within these dimensions.

All of this is also now detailed out in to begin to create what can only be called a unified field theory in Neuro-Semantics. Yet best of all, there is an immanently practical use of these four *meta-dimensions*.

They are practical for recognizing the *dimension* at which we're operating, for detecting the clues that indicate the different *dimensions,* developing elegant skill at working at each dimension of consciousness, discovering how to move up the dimensional hierarchy, and developing your felt sense of where you are with a client and what to do next.

The Meta-Levels within the Meta-Dimensions

Dimension I: The Representational Dimension

The first dimension involves what we select to represent on the screen of our mind. We do so in foregrounding some things while backgrounding others. We use our sensory representations to create our mental movie.

There are two meta-levels in this dimension. The first meta-level above that is *the editorial level* where we develop our style of working with the cinematic features of our movies (Sub-Modalities).

The next meta-level within this dimension involves linguistically representing the movies, labeling, classifying, categorizing, and all of the things we do with words (the Meta-Model of Language).

Basic meta-levels:
    1 Foreground - background
    2 Aware (awareness, cognizant)
    3 Think, thought (notion, idea, word)
    4 Feel, feeling
    5 So? Yes? And?
    6 Metaphor (story, poem, symbol)
    7 Open up, emerges
    8 Frame, framing
    9 Meaning
    10 See, sight, perceive
    11. Hear
    12. Say, Speak
    13. Refer, reference

Dimension II: The Meta-Stating Dimension

In this dimension we layer thoughts-and-emotions upon our representations. Here we set frames, via the mental-and-emotional states that we apply to our primary states. Our first-level beliefs are here which are warm, emotional, and full of conviction.

General meta distinctions —

14. Step back, witness
15. Meta, higher level
16. Transcend
17. Impress, Impression

Mental meta distinctions —

18. Believe, belief, confirm
19. Valid, validate, approve
20. Value, count, honor
21. Appreciate, celebrate
22. Permit, permission, allow, disconfirm, disallow
23. Prohibit, prohibition, taboo, censor
24. Disapprove
25. Resist, refusal
26. Decide, decision, choice, will
27. Weighing Pros and cons, oscillate
28. Conclude, conclusion
29. Intend, intention, will, desires
30. Outcome, goal, agenda
31. Interest, fascination
32. Expect, expectation
33. Anticipate, anticipation
34. Consequence, Consequential
35. Imply, implication
36. Differ, difference
37. Compare, comparison
38. Inspires, inspiration, moves
39. Ascribe, affix
40. Assess, assessment
41. Plan, game plan
42. Strategy, strategic
43. Connect, connection
44. Remember, memory, historical referent
45. Imagine, imagination, fantasy
46. Speculate, speculation
47. Judge, judgment
48. To know within self, conscience: should, must, ought
49. Converse, conversation
50. Reconcile, reconciliation
51. Insight, contemplate

52. Merit
53. Refer, reference, referent
54. Declare, declaration
55. Assert, assertion
56. Request, ask, implore
57. Narrate, narrative, story
58. Theater, play
59. Compute, computation
60. Punctuate, punctation
61. Bracket

Linguistic meta distinctions:
62. Catalogue, classify, group, encompass
63. Possible: can, could, will
64. Feasible: might, could
65. Probable, probability, extent, degree: might, may
66. Rules, demand, should
67. Author, authorize
68. Cause, causation
69. Define, definition, label
70. Class, classify
71. Category, categorize
72. Rubricize, rubric
73. Propose, proposal, proposition

Dimension III: The Gestalt Dimension

In this dimension, beliefs become belief-systems. There's much less emotional affect left, if any at all. And the state has been gestalted so that it works as a whole — commanding much more neurology. Installing states at this level requires meta-stating elegance for holding the gestalt as a whole while grounding it.

74. Generalize, generalization,
75. Abstract, abstraction
76. Construct, computation
77. Symbol, symbolize, symbolic
78. Realize, realization
79. Theme, thematic
80. Reason, rationale
81. Explain, explanation, exploratory

82. Extrapolate
83. Reckon, recognize
84. Reputation
85. Identity, identify, identification, self
86. Myth, archetype

Dimension IV: The Conceptual Dimension

In this dimension, the emotional quality drops out of the meta-states entirely. Here we experience our conceptual states as the sense of, "Of course." This represents a sense of reality as what we assume and expect. It's just "the way it is." With no emotion left, the experience seems purely "intellectual." Here we "know" what we know. Meta-states at this level are called concepts, principles, knowledge, reasons, models, paradigms, definitions.

87. Know, knowledge, epistemology
88. Abstract, abstraction
89. Principle
90. Conceive, concept
91. Presuppose, presupposition
92. Assume, assumption
93. Hypothesis, hypothesize
94. Propose, proposal, premise
95. Mathematize, mathematics
96. Equate, equation
97. Calculate, calculus, calculation
98. Understand, understanding
99. Comprehend, comprehension
100. Paradigm, model, map
101. Schema, schematize
102. Culture, cultivate

Others more recently found:
    Claim
    Purport
    Extrapolate
    Approve

THE | META- | DIMENSIONS

	Represent-ational	Meta-State	Gestalt	Conceptual
Mech-anisms	Repres. richness In all systems. Vividness Precise language Step in and out of your movies	Stepping back skill using reflexivity. Layering state upon state. Cognitive awareness of awareness.	Using repetition and intensity for Habituation. The coalescing of independent variables until a *whole* emerges	More habituation processes. Accepting as matter-of-fact assumptions.
Deframe in this dimension Dragons	Cinematic shifting Ecology Check Dragon Taming Movie Rewind New Behavior Generator	Quality Controlling Outframe with values, consequences Meta-state w/ negation Dragon Slaying / Transforming	Slowly unpeel Concept of meaning. Drop-Down Through Dancing w/ Dragons	"onion" Meta-state Challenge Fabric of Reality as a map. Dancing w/
Installing in this dimension	Become aware of representat. Sub-modality Shifts/ changes	Meta-stating pattern Apply resources to State Step back from Movie	Hold primary state and meta-state repeatedly. Gestalting pattern Open Up Belief System	Add repetition to Gestalting until reach "of course" state.

End Notes

1. In the Neuro-Logical Levels of Robert Dilts, his first three distinctions (behavior, capability, and environment) are not meta-levels but primary state levels. For more, see www.neurosemantics.com Articles: Meta-States, Logical Levels.

2. In Neuro-Semantics we speak about *the interfaces* of one state upon another and have identified 16 interfaces, see *Secrets of Personal Mastery* (1999) or the Training Manual, *Accessing Personal Genius.*

3. See *Mind-Lines* (2005, 5th edition). This book applies the Meta-Model distinctions to the skill of framing and reframing. Because lines can change minds, the discipline of reframing in 7 directions provides the structure of persuasion. This book updates the old outdated Sleight of Mouth patterns from NLP.

4. See the Meta-Coach Series, Volume I *Coaching Change* (2005) and Volume II *Coaching Conversations* (2006).

5. You can see this in the articles on www.neurosemantics.com that use the term "meta-domains" that refer to the 4 meta-models: Meta-Model of language, Meta-Programs, Meta-Modalities (sub-modalities), and Meta-States.

6. See *The Structure of Magic, Volume I and II,* also *User's Manual of the Brain, Volume I* which is an introduction to NLP.

7. See *The Secrets of Personal Mastery* (1999), *Meta-States* (1994/ 2000), and *NLP Going Meta* (2001).

8. This was the insightful discovery noted by Richard Bandler in *Using Your Brain — For a Change* (1985). Beliefs *command* the nervous system.

9. For more about the *Gestalting* pattern of resilience, see the chapter on Resilience in *Meta-States* (2000) or the Training Manual on *Resilience.*

10. See *Figuring Out People* (1997/ 2006) for an encyclopedia of meta-programs and a complete description of the Meta-Programs Model. Chapter Four describes meta-states as the source of meta-programs.

11. See *Using Your Brain — For a Change* (1985) as well as Andreas' work on sub-modalities. For an analysis of this, see *Sub-Modalities Going Meta.*

INDEX

Patterns

BIBLIOGRAPHY

Bandler, Richard; and Grinder, John. (1975, 1976). *The structure of magic, Volumes I and II: A book about language and therapy.* Palo Alto, CA: Science & Behavior Books.

Bains, Gurnek; Bains, Kylie. (2007). *Meaning Inc.: The blueprint for business success in the 21st century.* London, England: Profile Books Ltd.

Bannister, Dan; Fransella, Fay. (1971). *Inquiring man: The theory of personal constructs.* London: Penguin Books.

Bateson, Gregory. (1972). *Steps to an ecology of mind.* New York: Ballatine.

Beckwith, Harry. (1997). *Selling the invisible: A field guide to modern marketing.* New York: A Time Warner Company.

Blakeslee, Sandra; Blakeslee, Matthew. (2007). *The body has a mind of its own: How body maps in your brain help you do (almost) everything better.* NY: Random House.

Brothers, Chalmers. (2005). *Language and the pursuit of happiness.* Naples, FL: New Possibilities Press.

Bruner, Jerome. (1986). *Actual minds, possible worlds.* Cambridge, MA: Harvard University Press.

Bruner, Jerome. (1990). *Acts of meaning,* Cambridge, MA: Harvard University Press.

Carroll, John B. (Ed.) (1956). *Language, thought, and reality: Selected writings of Benjamin Lee Whorf.* New York: Wiley.

Chomsky, Noam. (1957). *Syntactic structures.* The Hague: Mouton Publishers.

Chomsky, Noam. (1965). *Aspects of the theory of syntax.* Cambridge, MA: MIT Press.

Csiksezentmihalyi, Mihaly. (1991). *Flow: The psychology of optimal experience.* New York: Harper & Row.

De Shazer, Steve (1991). *Putting difference to work.* New York: W.W. Norton & Company.

Dilts, Robert; Grinder, John; Bandler, Richard; DeLozier, Judith. (1980). *Neuro-linguistic programming, Volume I: The study of the structure of subjective experience.* Cupertino. CA.: Meta Publications.

Efran, Jay S.; Lukens, Michael D.; Lukens, Robert J.; *(1990). Language, structure and change: Frameworks of meaning in psychotherapy.* New York: W.W. Norton & Co.

Ellis, Albert. (1962). *Reason and emotion in psychotherapy.* New York: Lyle Stuart.

Ellis, Albert. (1973). *Humanistic psychotherapy: The rational-emotive approach.* New York: Julian Press.

Ellis, Albert and Harper, Robert A. (1976). *A new guide to rational living.* Englewood Cliffs, NJ: Prentice-Hall, Inc.

Fodor, Jerry A. (1987). *Psychosemantics: The problem of meaning in the philosophy of mind.* Cambridge: MIT Press.

Frankl, Viktor E. (1959). *Man's search for meaning: An introduction to logotherapy.* New York: Pocket Books.

Frankl, Viktor E. (1969). *The will to meaning: Foundations and applications of Logotherapy.* Middlesex, England: Penguin Books.

Frankl, Viktor E. (1978). *The unheard cry for meaning: Psychotherapy and humanism.* New York: Touchstone Book, Simon & Schuster.

Friedman, Steven (Ed.) (1993). *The new language of change: Constructive collaboration in psychotherapy.* New York: The Guilford Press.

Goffman, Erving. (1974). *Frame analysis: an essay on the organization of experience.* Cambridge MA: Harvard University Press.

Greenfield, Susan A. (1995). *Journey to the centers of the mind: Toward a science of consciousness.* New York: W. H. Freeman and Company.

Hall, L. Michael. (2007). *Meta-States: Managing the higher levels of your mind's reflexivity.* Clifton, CO: Neuro-Semantic Publications.

Hall, L. Michael; Bodenhamer, Bob G. (2005). *Sub-Modalities: Going Meta.* Formerly, The structure of Excellence. Clifton, CO: Neuro-Semantic Publications.

Hall, L. Michael. (2000). *Secrets of personal mastery: Advanced techniques for accessing your higher levels of consciousness. Wales, UK: Crown House Publications.*

Hall, L. Michael. (2001). *Communication Magic.* Wales, UK: Crown House Publications.

Hall, L. Michael; Duval, Michelle. (2004). *Coaching Conversations:* Robust Conversations that Coach for Excellence. Clifton, CO: Neuro-Semantic Publications.

Harris, Randy Allen. (1993). *The linguistic wars. NY: Oxford University Press.*

Heath, Chip; Heath, Dan. (2007). *Made to stick: Why some ideas survive and others die.* New York: Random House.

Jackendoff, Ray. (1994). *Patterns in the mind: Language and human nature.* New York: BasicBooks, Harper-Collins Publishers.

Johnson, Mark. (1987). *The body in the mind: The bodily basis of meaning, imagination, and reason.* Chicago: The University of Chicago Press.

Johnson, Mark. (2007). *The Meaning of the body: Aesthetics of Human Understanding.*

Kegan, Robert. (1994). *In over our heads: The mental demands of modern life. Cambridge, MA:* Harvard University Press.

Kelly, George A. (1955). *The psychology of personal constructs.* New York: Norton.

Korzybski, Alfred. (1933/1994). *Science and sanity: An introduction to non-Aristotelian systems and general semantics,* (5th. ed.). Lakeville, CN: International Non-Aristotelian Library Publishing Co.

Kuhn, Thomas S. (1970). *The structure of scientific revolutions* (2nd ed.). Chicago: University of Chicago Press.

Korzybski, Alfred (1949). Fate and freedom. In Lee, Irving, J. (Ed.). *The language of wisdom and folly.* New York: Harper & Brothers.

Korzybski, A. (1990). *Collected Writings: 0291-0591.* Kendig, M. and Read, C.S. (Eds.). Englewood, NJ: Institute of General Semantics.

Lakoff, George; Johnson, Mark. (1999). *Philosophy in the flesh: The embodied mind and its challenge to western thought.* NY: Basic Books.

Lakoff, George; Johnson, Mark. (1980). *Metaphors we live by.* Chicago, IL: The University of Chicago Press.

Lakoff, George. (1987). *Women, fire, and dangerous things: What categories reveal about the mind.* Chicago: The University of Chicago Press.

Langacker, Ronald. (1987). *Foundations of cognitive grammar,* Vol. 1. Stanford, CA: Stanford University Press.

Langacker, Ronald W. (1991). *Concept, image and symbol: The cognitive basis of grammar.* New York: Mouton de Gruyter.

Lenhardt, Vincent. (2004). *Coaching for meaning: The culture and practice of coaching and team building.* Translated by Malcolm Stewart. Macmillan: Palgrave.

Maslow, Abraham H. (1943). "A Theory of Human Motivation," *Psychological Review,* L, pp. 370-396. American Psychological Association.

Maslow, Abraham. (1970). *Motivation and Personality.* (2nd ed.). New York: Harper & Row.

Maslow, Abraham. (1968). *Toward a Psychology of Being.* New York: Van Nostrand.

Maslow, Abraham. (1953, 1971). *The Farther Reaches of Human Nature.* New York: Viking.

Mahoney, Michael J. (1991). *Human change processes: The scientific foundations of psychotherapy.* New York: BasicBooks.

Ogden, C.K.; Richards, I.A. (1923). *The meaning of meaning: A study of the influence of language upon thought and of the science of symbolism.* New York: A Harvest book, Harcourt, Brace & World, Inc.

Piaget, Jean. (1926). *The language and thought of the child.* New York: Harcourt Brace Jovanovich.

Piaget, Jean. (1954). *The construction of reality in the child.* Translated by Margaret Cook. New York: Basic Books.

Pinker, Stephen. (1997). *How the mind works.* New York: W.W. Norton & Co.

Polkinghorne, Donald. E. (1988). *Narrative knowing and the human sciences.* Albany, New York: State University of New York Press.

Scott, Susan. (2009). *Fierce Conversations: Achieving Success at work and in life, one conversation at a time.* New York: Viking.

Scott, Susan. (2009). *Fierce Leadership: A bold alternative to the worst "best" practices of business today.* New York: Broadway Business.

Steier, Frederick (Ed.) (1991). *Research and reflexivity.* Newbury Park, CA: Sage Publications.

Tournier, Paul. (1963). *Secrets.* Translated by Joe Embry, Richmond VA: John Knox Press.

Wadsworth, Barry J. (1989). *Piaget's theory of cognitive and affective development.* New York: Longman.

Wittgenstein, L. (1958). *The blue and brown books.* New York: Harper & Row.

Wittgenstein, L. (1968). *Philosophical investigations.* (G.E.M. Anscombe, trans.) (3rd Ed.). New York: Macmillan.

L. Michael Hall, Ph.D.

L. Michael Hall is a visionary leader in the field of NLP and Neuro-Semantics, and a modeler of human excellence. Searching out areas of human excellence, he models the structure of that expertise and then turns that information into models, patterns, training manuals, and books. With his several businesses, Michael is also an entrepreneur and an international trainer.

His doctorate is in the Cognitive-Behavioral sciences from Union Institute University. For two decades he worked as a psychotherapist in Colorado. When he found NLP in 1986, he studied and then worked with Richard Bandler. Later when studying and modeling resilience, he developed the Meta-States Model (1994) that launched the field of Neuro-Semantics. He co-created the *International Society of Neuro-Semantics* (ISNS) with Dr. Bob Bodenhamer. Learning the structure of writing, he began writing and has written more than 40 books, many best sellers in the field of NLP.

Applying NLP to coaching, he created the Meta-Coach System, this was co-developed with Michelle Duval (2003-2007), he co-founded the Meta-Coach Foundation (2003), created the Self-Actualization Quadrants (2004) and launched the new Human Potential Movement (2005).

Contact Information:
> P.O. Box 8
> Clifton, Colorado 81520 USA
> (1-970) 523-7877

Websites:
> www.neurosemantics.com
> www.meta-coaching.org
> www.self-actualizing.org
> www.meta-coachfoundation.org

Books by L. Michael Hall, Ph.D.

In NLP and Neuro-Semantics:

1) *Meta-States: Mastering the Higher Levels of Mind* (1995/ 2000).

2) *Dragon Slaying: Dragons to Princes* (1996 / 2000).

3) *The Spirit of NLP: The Process, Meaning and Criteria for Mastering NLP* (1996).

4) *Languaging: The Linguistics of Psychotherapy* (1996).

5) *Becoming More Ferocious as a Presenter* (1996).

6) *Patterns For Renewing the Mind* (with Bodenhamer, 1997 /2006).

7) *Time-Lining: Advance Time-Line Processes* (with Bodenhamer, 1997).

8) *NLP: Going Meta — Advance Modeling Using Meta-Levels* (1997/2001).

9) *Figuring Out People: Reading People Using Meta-Programs* (with Bodenhamer, 1997, 2005).

10) *SourceBook of Magic, Volume I* (with Belnap, 1997).

11) *Mind-Lines: Lines For Changing Minds* (with Bodenhamer, 1997/ 2005).

12) *Communication Magic* (2001). Originally, *The Secrets of Magic* (1998).

13) *Meta-State Magic: Meta-State Journal* (1997-1999).

14) *When Sub-Modalities Go Meta* (with Bodenhamer, 1999, 2005). Originally entitled, *The Structure of Excellence.*

15) *Instant Relaxation* (with Lederer, 1999).

16) *User's Manual of the Brain: Volume I* (with Bodenhamer, 1999).

17) *The Structure of Personality:* Modeling Personality Using NLP and Neuro-Semantics (with Bodenhamer, Bolstad, and Harmblett, 2001).

18) *The Secrets of Personal Mastery* (2000).

19) *Winning the Inner Game* (2007), originally *Frame Games* (2000).

20) *Games Fit and Slim People Play* (2001).

21) *Games for Mastering Fear* (with Bodenhamer, 2001).

22) *Games Business Experts Play* (2001).

23) *The Matrix Model: Neuro-Semantics and the Construction of Meaning* (2003).

24) *User's Manual of the Brain: Master Practitioner Course, Volume II* (2002).

25) *MovieMind: Directing Your Mental Cinemas* (2002).

26) *The Bateson Report* (2002).

27) *Make it So! Closing the Knowing-Doing Gap* (2002).

28) *Source Book of Magic, Volume II, Neuro-Semantic Patterns* (2003).

29) *Propulsion Systems* (2003).

30) *Games Great Lovers Play* (2004).

31) *Coaching Conversation, Meta-Coaching, Volume II* (with Michelle Duval & Robert Dilts 2004, 2010).

32) *Coaching Change, Meta-Coaching, Volume I* (with Duval, 2004).

33) *Unleashed: How to Unleash Potentials for Peak Performances* (2007).
34) *Achieving Peak Performance* (2009).
35) *Self-Actualization Psychology* (2008).
36) *Unleashing Leadership* (2009).
37) *The Crucible and the Fires of Change* (2010).
38) *Inside-Out Wealth* (2010).
39) *Benchmarking: The Art of Measuring the Unquantifiable* (2011).
40) *Innovations in NLP: Volume I* (Edited with Shelle Rose Charvet; 2011).
41) *Neuro-Semantics: Actualizing Meaning and Performance* (2011)

Other books:
1) *Emotions: Sometimes I Have Them/ Sometimes They have Me* (1985)
2) *Motivation: How to be a Positive Influence in a Negative World* (1987)
3) *Speak Up, Speak Clear, Speak Kind* (1987)
4) *Millennial Madness* (1992), now *Apocalypse Then, Not Now* (1996).
5) *Over My Dead Body* (1996).

Neuro-Semantics as an Association

In 1996 Hall and Bodenhamer registered "Neuro-Semantics" and founded *The International Society of Neuro-Semantics* (ISNS) as a new approach to teaching, training, and using NLP. The objective was to take NLP as a model and field to a higher level in terms of professional ethics and quality. Today Neuro-Semantics is one of the leading disciplines within NLP as it is pioneering many new developments and demonstrating a creativity that characterized NLP when it was new and fresh.

Dr. Hall is known as a prolific writer, having authored 41 books (2011) in the field of NLP and several others, many of them best sellers through *Crown House Publishes* (Wales, UK) and many of them translated into numerous languages: German, Dutch, Italian, Spanish, Russian, Japanese, Chinese, Arabic, Norwegian, Portuguese, etc.

www.neurosemantics.com
www.meta-coaching.org
www.metacoachingfoundation.org
www.self-actualizing.org

Order Books fro:

NSP: Neuro-Semantic Publications
P.O. Box 8
Clifton, CO. 81520—0008 USA
(970) 523-7877

Neuro-Semantic Trainings

Under the auspices of the International Society of Neuro-Semantics (ISNS), licensed Trainers train and certify NLP and Neuro-Semantic Trainings. See www.neurosemantics.com for more information and for a list of Neuro-Semantic Trainers and schedule of trainings.

NLP Trainings:

> *NLP Practitioner level:* Meta-NLP, intensive 7 to 12 days.
> *NLP Master Practitioner:* Meta-Masters, intensive 14 day training.

Neuro-Semantic Trainings:

> *Accessing Personal Genius* (APG)
> *Living Personal Genius*
> *Winning the Inner Game or Frame Games*
> *Learning Genius*
> *Defusing Hotheads*
> *Advanced Modeling Using Meta-Levels*
> *Advanced Flexibility Training*
> **NSTT: Neuro-Semantics NLP Trainers Training**

Business Trainings:

> *Games Business Experts Play*
> *Inside-Out Wealth*
> *Selling Excellence*
> *Mind-Lines*
> *Unleashing Leadership*

Health Training:

> *Games Slim and Fit People Play*
> *Resilience*
> *Neuro-Semantics of Health*
> *Unleashing Vitality*
> *Emotional Mastery*

Meta-Coaching Certification Training — www.meta-coaching.org

> *Coaching Essentials* (3 to 5 days)
> *Coaching Genius* (APG) (3 days).
> *Coaching Mastery* (for ACMC credentials, 8 days)
> *Professional Coach Certification* (PCMC, 10 days)
> *Master Coach Certification* (MCMC, 5 days)

Self-Actualization Trainings — www.self-actualizing.org

> *Unleashing Vitality*
> *Unleashing Potentials*
> *Unleashing Creativity Innovation*
> *Unleashing Leadership*

Neuro-Semantic Leaders

Joseph Scott and Jay Hedley — Australia
The Coaching Room Pty. Ltd.

Joseph and Jay are leading practitioners of Neuro-Semantics in the corporate space, specialising in Executive Coaching for individuals and Executive teams. In the public domain, specialising in coach training with the Meta-Coach Training System.
Level 29, Chifley Tower; Sydney, 2000, NSW, Australia
Phone: 1300 858 089
Email: joseph.scott@thecoachingroom.com.au
Web: http://www.thecoachingroom.com.au

Germaine Rediger — Belgium
InDialogue

Germaine Rediger offers a systematic approach to coaching in Neuro-Semantic trainings using cognitive-behavioral, developmental and self-actualization psychology as formulated in Neuro-Semantics. From this comes numerous practical tools for coaching and training which are ideally suited for CEO's, executives, managers, the international business and public sector context; a Licensed Trainer and Meta-Coach.
Rood Kruisstraat 48, 1500 Halle, Belgium
Phone: 00 32 2 305.35.45.   IPhone: +32 474 719469
germaine@indialogue.eu
Website: http://indialogue.eu

Mandy Chai — Hong Kong and China
Asia Professional Training Institute

Licensed Neuro-Semantics Trainer®; Associated Certified Meta-Coach®, Organizer of International Society of Neuro-Semantics — Greater China.
Mandy has an extensive background in delivering leading edge Self-Actualizing based Management Development and Organizational Transformation Programs for the last 15 years. She has taken the self-actualizing knowledge to a new level by applying them as the hub of all her training programs in cultural change, corporate excellence, team formation, leadership models. She enjoys organizing and working with individuals and organizations that want

to implement self-actualizing and change effectively, particularly when it involves the productivity and potential of people. She seeks to ensure the intellectual and emotional engagement of people and organizations to *Turn Vision into Reality.*

> Asia Professional Training Institute (www.apti.com.hk): mandy@apti.com.hk
> Talent Plus Corporate Training Consultant (www.talentplus.com.hk)
> International Society of Neuro-Semantics, Hong Kong and China (www.neurosemantics.com.hk)
> Address: 3/F, Tung Nam Commercial Centre, 42 Pitt Street, Yaumatei, Kowloon, Hong Kong
> Phones: (852) 27708886 (852) 96539667

Omar Salom — Mexico
Salom Change Dynamics

Omar has been a fountain of creativity with down-to-earth solutions for many companies. He has been working with many high potentials, CEOs and directors for the last 20 years, helping them to achieve higher results as they learn faster and take new challenges and for moving to higher positions.

> Psychologist and Executive Development Consultant; Licensed Neuro-Semantic Trainer
> Omar@salomchd.com; www.salomchd.com
> Cell Phone: 5215-5 919- 96329 (Mexico City)
> Office: 5255 -3093-0686 /3093- 0687

David Murphy — Mexico

The constant search for answers on how people are successful in their lives and how they manage to live in the fullness of resources, has led David to study NLP and Neuro-Semantics the last 10 years to the point of becoming a member of the International Leadership Team. David is Trainer and consultant in NLP, Neuro-Semantics Models and (PCMC) Professional Certified Meta-Coach.

> david@neurosemantica-latam.com;
> neurosemantica@hotmail.com; contact@davidmurphy.mx;
> Web site: www.davidmurphy.mx
> Phone: +52-967-679-06-66; Office: +52-967-674-71-38

Alan Fayter, DCH (Distinction) — New Zealand

Optimum Mind Ltd

Neuro-Semantic and NLP coach and trainer; based in New Zealand, Alan coaches and trains to ISNS and IANLP standards worldwide. He uses practical, performance based methods to help executives, leadership teams and individuals perform to their highest potentials.
Phone: +64 03.942 2103
www.optimum-mind.co.nz
alan@optimum-mind.co.nz

Colin Cox and Lena Gray — New Zealand

Ignition Training Systems

0800 17 0111
120/3 Nelson Crescent, Napier,
New Zealand
colin@ignition.org.nz; lena@ignition.org.nz
www.ignition.org.nz

Lene Fjellheim — Norway

CoachTeam

CoachTeam has two primary focuses: 1) Coach Academy: One is to be the leading school in Norway in training and development of managers and coaches. Students are certified after International ABNLP with ISNS standard. 2) Corporate programs, coaching, workshops, courses and lectures in communication, motivation, team building, ethics and international leadership programs. She is a Licensed NLP/Neuro-Semantic Trainer; PCMC Credentialed Meta-Coach.
P. O. Box 4440, Nydalen, 0403 Oslo, Norway
www.coachteam.no
www.coachakademiet.no
Lene@coachteam.no

Tim Goodenough — South Africa

Coaching Unity International
tim@coachingunity.co.za; www.coachingunity.co.za

Cheryl Lucas and Carey Jooste — South Africa
People SA Coaching · Leadership

Cheryl and Carey are Licensed Meta Coach Trainers®, International Neuro Semantic Trainers and Professional Certified Meta Coaches (PCMC). Their passion and focus is Actualizing Excellence in Individuals, Teams, and Organisations.
cheryl@psacoaching.co.za
carey@psacoaching.co.za
Tel: +27 12 362 6542; Fax: +27 12 362 3167
www.psacoaching.co.za

Femke Stuut MSC.— United States
The Pepper Plant

With an unbridled compassion for people and the power of their dreams and an incurable habit of turning rocks over, Femke Stuut stands out as an inspiring coach and trainer. She is an architect of intellectual awareness, personal and cultural transformation with proven abilities to unearth missions, values and goals and make reality of them.
Executive and Cultural Development Consultant
Licensed Neuro-Semantics Trainer and Meta-Coach
femke@getpeppered.com
Cell phone: +1 (415) -623 -9286